INTERMITTENT FASTING FOR WOMEN OVER 50

Discover How to Lose Weight, Delay Aging and Enhance Your Energy to Regain Your Best Shape in Your 50's | BONUS 50 Recipes and 21-Day Meal Plan

Aileen Terry

Table of Contents

Introduction

Fasting is an ancient practice that has been practiced by many cultures and religions, such as Islam's month-long Ramadan or the Jewish Yom Kippur. In a nutshell, intermittent fasting means not ingesting any calories for extended periods. While most people think of this as abstaining from all food and liquid, it can also consist of restricting calorie intake on certain days, which is called intermittent fasting.

It has been found to have many benefits for both men and women: improved weight loss, better blood sugar control, increased focus, improved skin complexion, weight maintenance, reduced anxiety, depression, and blood pressure.

Intermittent fasting is particularly effective for older adults as it helps improve insulin sensitivity which promotes healthy metabolism and helps the body better utilize blood sugar.

Intermittent fasting is also great for hormonal health. By helping optimize insulin sensitivity and blood sugar levels, your hormones can run more efficiently. This includes helpful hormones like leptin, which help manage your appetite, and ghrelin, which stimulates your body's hunger response. These hormones are critical in managing weight by getting you into a healthy calorie-burning balance.

Women and Intermittent Fasting

There are different types of intermittent fasting, yet it is most effective if done daily. One of the ways that women can do this is to have a fast day and eat according to their body's needs. Does this sound like you?

A fast day means you have one day where you don't eat any food or drink anything but water. You might consider fasting every other day, alternating with non-fast days, where you eat as much as feels good for your body. How long should these fasting days be? It can vary based on how clean your diet has been and how many calories that meal the previous day has. Ideally, it will be from 10 to 14 hours. The general recommendation is not to go over 16 hours.

As you can imagine, older women may find fasting difficult and should consult their health care practitioner before trying any form of fasting. Women who are pregnant or breastfeeding should also consult their physician before trying a fast day.

Remember, this is not an extreme form of fasting. The goal is to simply help you realize how you feel when you are not eating or drinking anything. You may be surprised at the benefits of a 10-12-hour fast day.

This type of intermittent fasting will also show you how much food is truly necessary for sustaining yourself daily. You can then work to incorporate and minimize your food intake while still eating the foods you enjoy.

Keep this in mind, however: the results of fasting do not come from skipping a meal or eating less. They come from changing to a healthier lifestyle that includes healthier foods and portion sizes.

Another great way to get some of the benefits of fasting is simply restricting your calorie intake on a given day. This can be done by restricting your daily calorie intake by 20 percent. While this is more than what most experts recommend, it may be the perfect kick-start to your weight loss journey if you are already eating well and working out regularly.

The first fast day in this protocol is generally done one to two weeks after the beginning of your weight loss journey. This way, if you are already on a meal plan, you will soon be able to begin incorporating fasting into your lifestyle. If you are not on a meal plan, I recommend consulting with your health care professional before starting the intermittent fasting protocol.

Chapter 1. What Is Intermittent Fasting

In the first place, we should get a smidgen of foundation data on how and why individuals even think to utilize this strategy. A few groups accept that eating less or fasting discontinuously assists them with getting thinner simpler by diminishing their "calorie admission while keeping up with supplement thickness."

Others feel that irregular fasting can help them stay better by diminishing the measure of insulin, which is a chemical that permits you to convey glucose from your blood to the cells. In conclusion, numerous individuals trust it's simply a great method to work on their general wellbeing and prosperity. So how does the entirety of this work?

Indeed, when eating dinners or doing irregular fasting, we are, as a rule, in what is known as a "took care of state" because the food you eat is giving glucose or sugar to your body to utilize. At the point when you're in taken care of the state, you are invigorating the creation of insulin, which is the chemical that empowers you to convey glucose from your blood to the cells.

Discontinuous fasting hinders insulin emission and restrains your body's capacity to store fat. This is because when we eat, insulin impedes lipolysis (the cycle through which muscle to fat ratio is separated into free unsaturated fats), so it permits your body to retain abundant sugar from your circulation system.

After a time of not eating, in any case, insulin and glucose levels drop. This creates an "anabolic" climate for building muscle and losing muscle to fat ratio. During fasting, lipolysis is expanded because of the centralization of unsaturated fats in the circulatory system increments. What's the significance here?

It implies that fat cells separate into more modest unsaturated fats, which are then delivered into the circulatory system to be utilized by the muscles as energy! Anyway, what does this all mean? It basically implies that you can make an anabolic state for building muscle and losing muscle to fat ratio while fasting by having your glucose level dip under a specific limit (generally around 70). There are a couple of various ways to deal with this; however, the 16/8 technique is the most well-known. With this technique, you would quickly for 16 hours of the day and eat for 8 hours afterwards. So, if you get up at 7 in the morning, you cannot eat again until later that night at 9 pm.

Another way to do it is 8/16 or 12/12. The difference between these two methods is when your daily fast begins and ends.

This is because it's more effective for fat loss and muscle gain than the other two methods. However, if you really prefer the 12/12 or 8/16 method, then do that instead. I don't recommend trying all three methods at once because your results won't be as clear when you're not consistently sticking to one method.

Intermittent Fasting for Women Over 50

Intermittent fasting can help improve your health and body composition, but the key is not to overdo it. It will be fine if you follow it for a couple of days a week—maybe even four times per week. But if you try to do it every single day, then that's how you can end up harming your body.

The first few days are going to be tough. Really tough! But you have to push through, and I promise that you will feel amazing when those first few days are done! As a result, begin slowly and gradually increase your workload. You would be overjoyed that you did!

There are a few important rules to remember when fasting:

- It's best to stop eating at least 3 hours before you go to bed. This is important for a few reasons. First, while you sleep, your body is busy burning fat. You don't want to slow down that process by eating just before bedtime. Second, while you sleep, your body uses its glycogen stores as an energy source, and the last thing you want is for those stores to run too low (which can cause muscle wasting).
- Don't exercise too late in the day. You can go on a walk in the morning or go to the gym in the afternoon, but don't do anything too strenuous later on in the day.
- Don't eat too close to bedtime. I know that you probably want to pack in as many calories as possible, and if you fall asleep after eating a big meal,
- Don't confuse skipping meals with intermittent fasting. If there is an event or something that you need to eat a little extra, then, by all means, do so. Just don't make a habit of it.
- Don't push your body too hard. If you're lifting weights in the morning, then go really easy on yourself for the rest of the day.

Chapter 2. How does Intermittent Fasting Works?

Intermittent fasting is the technique of scheduling your dishes for your body to obtain the most out of them. Rather than minimizing your calorie use by 50%, refuting yourself of all the foods you value, or diving right into a classy diet plan pattern, intermittent fasting is an all-natural, logical, and also balanced method of eating that advertises fat burning. There are tons of ways to approach Intermittent Fasting.

It's defined as an eating pattern. This technique focuses on altering what you take in instead of what you consume.

When you begin Intermittent fasting, you will be more than likely to maintain your calorie intake the same; nonetheless, in contrast to spreading your dishes throughout the day, you will undoubtedly eat more significant recipes throughout a much shorter amount of time. For example, as opposed to consuming 3 to 4 meals a day, you might eat one big meal at 11 am, afterwards an added large dish at 6 pm, without any dine-in between 11 am as well as 6 pm, as well as also after 6 pm, no meal up until 11 am the adhering to day. This is simply one strategy of recurring fasting, and likewise, others will be examined in this book in later stages.

Intermittent Fasting is a technique many bodybuilders, specialist athletes, and physical health and fitness masters use to maintain their muscular tissue mass high and their body fat percent reduced. Recurring fasting can be short-term or long-term, but the best results originate from embracing this technique right into your everyday lifestyle.

For 3 to 5 hours after consuming a meal, your body remains in what is described as the "fed state." Your insulin levels rise throughout the fed state to soak up and digest your meal. When your insulin levels get high, it is exceptionally tough for your body to shed fat. Insulin is a hormone produced by the pancreatic to handle sugar degrees in the bloodstream. Its purpose is to manage insulin as technically a hormonal storage agent. When insulin degrees become so high, your body starts shedding your food for energy instead of your conserved fat. This is why boosted degrees protect against weight reduction.

After the 3 to 5 hrs are up, your body has finished refining the dish, and also you enter the post-absorptive state. The post-absorptive state lasts anywhere from 8 to 12 hours. When your body comes, hereafter, the time room is the fasted state as a result of the reality that your body has refined your food by this.

Factor, your insulin levels are reduced, making you keep fat extremely available for losing.

Persisting fasting allows your body to get to an innovative weight loss state that you would usually obtain with the average' 3 meals daily' eating pattern. They are just altering the timing as well as the pattern of their food intake. When you start an Intermittent Fasting program right into the swing of points, it may take some time. Merely obtain back if you slip up right into your Intermittent fasting pattern when you can.

Making a way of living entails a purposeful initiative, and no one expects you to do it completely today. Intermittent fasting will take some getting used to if you are not in the practice of going long periods without eating. As long as you pick the right technique for you, remain focused, and remain concentrated, you will unanimously grasp it quickly.

Unlike some of the other diet regimen strategies you may embark on, the Intermittent fast will certainly work. It is simple to obtain a bit terrified regarding fasting when you listen to it.

Recurring fasting is a little bit various than you might assume. If you finish up being on, your body will often go right into hunger mode, the rapid for as well lengthy.

You do not need to get concerned about exactly how this Intermittent will quickly work in the craving's mode. The Intermittent fast is efficient because you are not going too quickly for as long as the body gets in right into this malnourishment setting and stops minimizing weight. Instead, it will make the rapid continue long enough that you will have the ability to accelerate the metabolic process.

With the Intermittent quick, you will discover that when you opt for a couple of hrs. Without eating (usually no more than 2 - 4 hrs.), the body is not going to go right into a malnourishment setting. When complying with a recurring fasting plan, you require your body to melt more fat without placing it in any sort of extra job.

Here Are a Couple of Fast Pointers for Success

Mostly, it is essential not to expect to see outcomes from your new lifestyle promptly. Perhaps, you need to focus on devoting yourself to the process for a minimum of 30 days before starting to evaluate the results correctly.

Second, it is imperative to remember that the excellent quality of the food you place into your body still matters. It will certainly merely take a few convenience food meals to reverse all of your tough work.

For excellent results, you will plan to consist of an in-light exercise routine during quick days along with a far more fundamental regimen for full-calorie days.

Recurring Fasting describes nutritional consumption patterns that include not consuming or continues limiting calories for a long-term period, Intermittent Fasting (IF). There are various subgroups of regular fasting, each with variance in the fast of individuals, some for hours, others for day(s). This has finished up being an extremely liked subject in the clinical research area as a result of every one of the prospective advantages of fitness in addition to health that is being found.

The diet regimen you adhere to whilst Recurring Fasting will be figured out by the results you are looking for and where you are beginning with additionally, so take a look at it on your own and ask the question, what do I want from this?

If you are looking to lose a significant quantity of weight, then you are misting likely to have to take a look at your diet regimen plan extra closely, yet if you wish to shed a couple of pounds for the beach, then you could discover that a pair of weeks of Recurring fasting can do that for you.

There are many various ways you can do recurring fasting. We are most likely to consider the 24-hour fasting system, which is what I used to shed 27 pounds over a 2-month duration. You could really feel some cravings pains, but these will also pass. As you end up being even more familiar with Intermittent fasting, you might find, as I have that feeling of need no more existing you with a concern.

Suppose you are fretted that you are not getting adequate nutrients into your body. In that case, you might consider a juice made from celery, lime, broccoli, and ginger, which will taste fantastic and get some sufficient nutrients fluid into your body.

Whatever your diet strategy is, whether it's healthy or not, you should see weight reduction after three weeks of intermittent fasting. Do not be put off if you do not find much advancement at first. It's not a race, and also, it is much, far better to drop weight in a straight style over time as opposed to collision losing a couple of extra pounds, which you will put right back on. After the initial month, you might want to look at your diet plan on non-fasting days and remove high sugar foods and even any scrap that you might generally take in. I have discovered that intermittent fasting over the long term tends to make me wish to consume healthier foods as an all-natural routine.

Suppose you are practicing intermittent fasting for bodybuilding. In that case, you may wish to consider looking at your macro-nutrients and also working out just how much healthy protein and carbohydrate you call for to eat. This is a lot more complex, as well as you can also uncover info about this on several websites that you will need to spend time examining for the very best end results.

There are great deals of advantages to recurring fasting, which you will view as you proceed. A few of these advantages include even more energy, much less bloating, a clearer mind, and a basic feeling of wellness. It's important not to succumb to any lure to binge eat after a fasting duration, as this will negate the influence obtained from the recurring fasting period.

In verdict, simply by adhering to two times a week 24-hour Intermittent Fasting approach for a couple of weeks, you will slim down; however, if you can boost your diet plan on the days that you do not fast, then you will lose more weight, and if you can remain with this system, then you will certainly keep the weight off without turning to any kind of fad diet regimen or diet plans that are difficult to stick to.

Chapter 3. Types of Intermittent Fasting

16/8 Method

This is just about the most popular fasting method since it's so schedule-based, meaning there are no surprises. Based on your everyday life, this will give you the freedom to control when you eat. Sixteen is the number of hours you're likely to be fasting, which may also be lowered to twelve or perhaps fourteen hours if that better fits into your life. Then, your eating period will be between eight and ten hours every day. This might seem daunting, but it just means that you are skipping an entire meal. Many people choose to begin their fast around 7 or 8 pm and then not eat until 11 or noon the next day, which means they fast for the recommended 16 hours. Of course, it isn't as bad as it sounds since they are sleeping during this time, so it comes down to eating dinner and then not eating again until the next day around lunch, so you are just skipping breakfast.

You will be doing it every day, so it is important to find the hours that work for you. If you work the third shift, switching your eating period around to fit into your schedule is important. If you find yourself being run down and sluggish, tweak your fasting hours until you find a healthy balance. Granted, there will be some adjustment because chances are your body is not accustomed to skipping entire meals. However, this should go away after a couple of weeks. If it doesn't, try starting your fasting period earlier in the day, allowing you to eat earlier the next, or alter it however you need to feel healthy and happy.

Lean-Gains Method (14:10)

The lean-gains method has several different incarnations on the web, but its fame comes from the fact that it helps shed fat while building it into muscle almost immediately. Through the lean-gains method, you'll find yourself able to change all that fat into muscle through a rigorous practice of fasting, eating right, and exercising.

Through this method, you fast anywhere from 14 to 16 hours and spend the remaining 10 or 8 hours each day engaged in eating and exercising. Unlike the crescendo, this method features daily fasting and eating rather than alternating days of eating versus not. Therefore, you don't have to be quite cautious about extending the physical effort to exercise on the days you are fasting because those days when you're fasting are every day!

For the lean-gaining method, start fasting only for 14 hours and work it up to 16 if you feel comfortable with it, but never forget to drink enough water and be careful about spending too much energy on exercise! Remember that you want to grow in health and potential through intermittent fasting. You'll certainly not want to lose any of that growth by forcing the process along.

20:4 Method

Stepping things up a notch from the 14:10 and 16:8 methods, the 20:4 method is tough to master, for it is rather unforgiving. People talk about this method of intermittent fasting as intense and highly restrictive. Still, they also say that the effects of living this method are almost unparalleled by all other tactics.

For the 20:4 method, you'll fast for 20 hours each day and squeeze all your meals, eating, and snacking into 4 hours. People who attempt 20:4 normally have two smaller meals or just one large meal and a few snacks during their 4-hour window to eat, and it is up to the individual which four hours of the day they devote to eating.

The trick for this method is to make sure you're not overeating or bingeing during those 4-hour windows to eat. It is all-too-easy to get hungry during the 20-hour fast and have that feeling propel you into intense and unrealistic hunger or meal sizes after the fast period is over. Be careful if you try this method. If you're new to intermittent fasting, work your way up to this one gradually, and if you're working your way up already, only make the shift to 20:4 when you know you're ready. It would surely be disappointing if all your progress with intermittent fasting got hijacked by one poorly thought-out goal with the 20:4 method.

Meal Skipping

Meal skipping is an extremely flexible form of intermittent fasting that can provide all of the benefits of intermittent fasting but with less strict scheduling. If you are not on a typical schedule or feel like a stricter variation of the intermittent fasting diet will serve you, meal skipping is a viable alternative.

Many people who choose to use meal skipping find it a great way to listen to their bodies and follow their basic instincts. If they are not hungry, they simply don't eat that meal. Instead, they wait for the next one. Meal skipping can also help people who have time constraints and who may not always be able to get in a certain meal of the day.

It is important to realize that you may not always maintain a 10-16-hour window of fasting with meal skipping. As a result, you may not get every benefit from other fasting diets. However, this may be an excellent solution for people who want an intermittent fasting diet that feels more natural. It may also be a great idea for those looking to begin listening to their bodies more so that they can adjust to a more intense variation of the diet with greater ease. It can be a great transitional diet for you if you are not ready to jump into one of the other fasting diets just yet.

Warrior Diet Fasting

The most extreme form of intermittent fasting is known as the Warrior Diet. This intermittent fasting cycle follows a 20-hour fasting window with a short 4-hour eating window. During that eating window, individuals are supposed only to consume raw fruits and vegetables. They can also eat one large meal. Typically, the eating window occurs at night time to snack throughout the evening, have a large meal, and then resume fasting.

Because of the length of fasting during the Warrior Diet, people should also consume a fairly hearty level of healthy fats. Doing so will give the body something to consume during the fast to produce energy with. A small number of carbohydrates can also be incorporated to support energy levels too.

People who eat the Warrior Diet tend to believe that humans are natural nocturnal eaters and that we are not meant to eat throughout the day. The belief is that eating this way follows our natural circadian rhythms, allowing our bodies to work optimally.

The only people who should consider doing the Warrior Diet are those who have already had success with other forms of intermittent fasting and are used to it. Attempting to jump straight into the Warrior Diet can have serious repercussions for anyone who is not used to intermittent fasting. Even still, those who are used to it may find this particular style too extreme for them to maintain.

Eat-Stop-Eat (24 Hour) Method

This method of fasting is incredibly similar to the crescendo method. The only discernable difference is that there's no anticipation of increasing into a more intense fasting pattern with time. For the eat-stop-eat method, you decide which days you want to take off from eating, and then you run with it until you've lost that weight, and keep running with the lifestyle for good because you won't be able to imagine life without it.

The eat-stop-eat method involves one to two days a week being 100% oriented towards fasting, with the other five to six days concerning "business as normal." The one or two days spent fasting are then full 24-hour days spent without eating anything at all. These days, of course, water and coffee are still fine to drink, but no food items can be consumed whatsoever. Exercise is also frowned upon on those fasting days, but see what your body can handle before deciding how that should all work out.

Some people might start thinking they're using the crescendo method but end up sticking with eat-stop-eat.

Alternate-Day Method

The alternate-day method is admittedly a little confusing, but the reason it could be so confusing could come, in part, from how much wiggle room it provides for the practitioner. This method is great for people who don't have a consistent schedule or any sense of one, it is incredibly forgiving for those who don't quite have everything together for themselves yet.

When it comes down to it, alternate-day intermittent fasting is really up to you. You should try to fast every other day, but it doesn't have to be that precise. Similarly, with the crescendo method, you're set as long as you fast two to three days a week, with a break day or two in between each fasting day! Then, you'll want to eat normally for three or four days out of each week, and when you encounter a fasting day, you don't even need to fast completely!

Alternate-day fasting is a solid place to start, especially if you work a varying schedule or still have yet to get used to a consistent one. If you want to make things more intense from this starting point, the alternate-day method can easily become the eat-stop-eat, crescendo, or the 5:2 method. Essentially, this method is a great place to begin

12:12 Method

As another of the more natural ways of intermittent fasting, the 12:12 approach is well-suited for beginning practitioners. Of course, many people live out the 12:12 method without any forethought simply because of their sleeping and eating schedule, but turning the 12:12 into a conscious practice can have just as many positive effects on your life as the more drastic 20:4 method claims.

According to a study conducted at the University of Alabama, for this method, in particular, you fast for 12 hours and then enter a 12-hour eating window. With this method, it's not difficult whatsoever to get three small meals and several snacks or two big meals and a snack into your day. With the 12:12, the standard meal timing works just fine.

Ultimately, this method is a great one to start from, for a lot of variation can be built into this scheduling when you're ready to make things more interesting. For example, effortlessly and without much effort, 12:12 can become 14:10 or even 16:8, and in seemingly no time, you can find yourself trying alternate-day or crescendo methods. So start with what's normal for you, and this method might be exactly that!

5:2 Method

This is another popular way to fast because there is no true fasting involved, but instead, a strict and drastic calorie reduction for two days each week. So, you will eat your normal 1,600 to 2,000 calories and exercise like normal for five days a week. On two non-consecutive days a week, you will restrict your caloric intake to between 500 and 600 calories. When doing this, pay close attention to the number of calories in beverages as well; many people make the mistake of only counting calories in what they eat. Remember that beverages contain calories, too, especially if you are drinking things from coffee shops, as these tend to have high amounts of sugar.

Chapter 4. Benefits of Intermittent Fasting for Women Over 50 Years Old

There are plenty of diets, all promising you the impossible—incredible weight loss, with no mention of any side effects. You are probably fed up with the "lose X pounds in 30 days, guaranteed" approach. Unfortunately, many of these diets are not backed up by science. Or in other words, there is no scientific research to prove these diets deliver what they promise. Instead, they focus only on the weight loss process, suggesting meal plans that are incredibly radical in some cases.

Diets mean nutrient deprivation in most cases, but they are plenty of instances where these diets have harmful effects on your health. Unlike other diets, focusing on the weight loss process in an incredibly short amount of time, intermittent fasting focuses more on your health. Nutritionists believe that fitness should be the most crucial factor. Only a healthy body can have a long and sustainable weight loss process; unlike the other diets, which have a "hit and run" approach, IF is something for the long run and should be regarded as a way of life, not like a meal plan to be implemented for a few weeks. By checking out the benefits below, you can better understand why this process is beneficial for your body.

The main benefits of intermittent fasting can be summarized in 8 points:

1. Eliminates precancerous and cancerous cells.
2. Shifts quickly into nutritional ketosis.
3. Reduces the fat tissue.
4. Enhances the gene expression for healthspan and longevity.
5. Induces autophagy and the apoptotic cellular repair or cleaning.
6. Improves your insulin sensitivity.
7. Reduces inflammation and oxidative stress.
8. Increase neuroprotection and cognitive effects.

To expand on the benefits of this practice, intermittent fasting can have positive impacts on the fat loss process, disease prevention, anti-aging, therapeutic benefits (psychological, spiritual, and physical), mental performance, physical fitness (improved metabolism, wind, and endurance, the significant effect over bodybuilding).

Healthy Eating Habits

As you restrain yourself from eating, the body will no longer have available glucose to use to produce energy. Therefore, it will use ketones to break the fat tissue open and release the energy stored. That is how the body will burn your existing fat to generate power. However, they are not designed for the long run for diets, and as soon as you break the diet, you will start gaining weight again. Intermittent fasting is something you can try for a lifetime because it is easy to stick to, and it doesn't involve any particular meal plan. You can eat your favorite food as long as you schedule your meals, allowing a smaller eating window and a more extended fasting period IF induces ketosis and eventually autophagy, which will reduce the fat reserves.

Preventing Diseases

What if you found out that intermittent fasting is, in fact, a cure for several different diseases and medical conditions? You would become more interested in this process. A few studies show the beneficial effects IF has on your health. For example, patients with type 2 diabetes who follow a short-term regular intermittent fasting regimen have lower body weight and higher post-meal glucose variability, according to research published in the World Journal of Diabetes.

Other benefits this diet has are:

- Enhances the markers of stress resistance
- Reduces the blood pressure and inflammation
- Better lipid levels and glucose circulation may lead to a lower risk of cardiovascular disease, neurological diseases like Parkinson's and Alzheimer's, and cancer.

Anti-Aging Process

The modern-day lifestyle is excessively stressful and sedentary. Whether we like it or not, these variables play a significant role in the aging process. You probably think what, if anything, intermittent fasting can do to slow down this operation, which we all know can't be prevented. IF isn't a "fountain of youth," and it won't make you immortal. However, it can lower blood pressure, reduce oxidative damage, enhance insulin sensitivity, and reduce fat mass. Coincidence or not, these factors are known to improve your health and longevity. Intermittent fasting is one of the triggering factors of autophagy, a process known for destroying and replacing old cell parts with new ones at any level within your body. Such an approach can slow down the aging process.

Therapeutic Benefits

Physical, spiritual, and psychological benefits are the most significant clinical benefits. Intermittent fasting is a powerful diabetes remedy in terms of physical benefits. However, it can be very helpful in reducing seizure-related brain damage and seizures and improving arthritis symptoms. This practice has spiritual significance since it is commonly used for religious purposes all over the world. While some practitioners regard fasting as penance, it is also a practice for purifying the body and soul (according to the theological apologist).

Intermittent fasting is also about exercising control and will over your body and your feelings. Achieving absolute control over your power and mind is a compelling psychological benefit. For example, you can ignore hunger and restrain yourself from eating for a certain period. In other words, IF is also associated with mind training and can also improve your self-esteem. A successful intermittent fasting regime can have potent effects from a psychological point of view. A study has shown that women practicing IF had terrific results regarding senses of control, reward, pride, and achievement.

Brain Health

IF also enhances cognitive function and is very useful for boosting your brainpower. This argument can be supported by several factors related to intermittent fasting. To begin with, it raises the amount of brain-derived neurotrophic factor (BDNF), a protein in the brain that interacts with the parts of the brain that regulate cognitive and memory functions and learning.

Even new brain cells can be protected and stimulated by BDNF. You will reach the ketogenic state via IF, in which your body uses ketones to convert fat into energy. Ketones can also nourish your brain, improving mental acuity, efficiency, and energy levels.

Improved Physical Fitness

This process influences not only your brain but also your digestive system. Setting a small feeding window and a more significant fasting period will encourage the proper digestion of food. That leads to a balanced and healthy daily intake of food and calories. The more you get used to this process, the less you will experience hunger. If you are worried about slowing your metabolism, think again! IF enhances your metabolism, it makes metabolism more flexible, as the body can now run on glucose or fats for energy in a very effective way. In other words, intermittent fasting leads to better metabolism.

Oxygen use during exercise is a crucial part of the success of your training. You simply cannot have performance without adjusting your breathing habits during workouts. VO2 max represents the maximum amount of oxygen your body can use per minute or kilogram of body weight. In popular terms, VO2 max is also referred to as "wind." The more oxygen you use, the better you will be able to perform. Top athletes can have twice the VO2 level of those without any training. A study focused on the VO2 levels of a fasted group (they just skipped breakfast) and a non-fasted group (they had breakfast 1 hour before). For both groups, the VO2 level was at 3.5 L./min. In the beginning and after the study, the level showed a significant increase of "wind" for the fasting group (9.7%), compared to just a 2.5% increase in the case of those with breakfast.

Bodybuilding

Having a narrow feeding window automatically means fewer meals to concentrate the daily calorie intake into just 1–2 consistent meals. Bodybuilders find this approach a lot more pleasing than having the same calorie consumption split into 5–6 different meals throughout the day. It is said that you need a specific number of proteins just to maintain your muscle mass. However, muscle mass can also be supported through intermittent fasting, a process that doesn't focus specifically on protein intake. Remember, the growth hormone reaches unbelievable levels after 48 hours of fasting, so you can easily maintain your muscles without eating many proteins or having protein bars or shakes.

As you already know, nothing is perfect and intermittent fasting is no exception. There are a few side effects that you need to worry about, like:

- Hunger is perhaps the most common side effect of this way of eating, but the more you get used to IF, the less hunger you will feel.
- Beware of constipation, as when you eat less, you will not have to go to the toilet very often, so you can feel constipated at the beginning.
- Headaches should be expected when fasting. Food deprivation is a direct cause of these headaches. However, controlling your hunger and getting used to fasting will be the best weapon to fight against these headaches.
- You might experience muscle cramps, heartburn, and dizziness during intermittent fasting.
- In the case of athletic women or those with deficient body fat percentage, intermittent fasting may lead to a higher risk of irregular periods and lower chances of conception (so it reduces fertility for these women).

Chapter 5. Why Intermittent Fasting for Women Over 50?

Cell Regeneration, Longevity, and Immunity

When we age, our body's innate capacity to fight off contamination and cell recovery decrease as connected to age. In basic terms, it implies when we are defied with a disease, particularly gastrointestinal ones, it takes us longer to recuperate.

At the point when an individual diet, we control our calorie admission, and researchers have asserted that a lower admission of calories is straightforwardly connected to life span. Foundational microorganisms are a critical piece of our wellbeing, as they fix any harm happening inside and remotely to the body.

When we quick, it triggers our "metabolic switch" that boots the level at which our bodies recover their cells. These progressions on a cell level are something noteworthy to have the option to control, and fasting just improves our capacity to do as such.

Heart Health

A lot of examination is being finished concerning heart wellbeing and the effect that irregular fasting has on it. Results look encouraging and show that discontinuous fasting can be one of the principal instruments to diminish our coronary illness hazard.

One of the fundamental reasons individuals show better well-being when fasting is that they practice a degree of control in counting calories and exercise. This thought of upkeep prompts losing over into their customary dietary patterns, in any event, when they are not fasting. Both eating regimen and exercise demonstrate once more to be fundamental while staying away from any type of ailment.

Fasting likewise controls your glucose and cholesterol levels, the two elements which sway your probability of causing coronary illness or encountering a cardiovascular failure. Fasting diminishes the degree of "awful" cholesterol - lipoprotein - in your circulation system and oversees how our bodies process sugar.

Controlling these two components assists us with trying not to foster kind two diabetes and corpulence, the two of which are two contributing elements while referencing coronary illness.

Circadian Rhythm

Circadian rhythm, and what makes it mean for you? The circadian rhythm is the interaction that happens inside your body to manage your rest and wake cycles. This cycle rehashes at regular intervals. Our bodies have gotten used to eating during and resting around evening time throughout the long term. Notwithstanding, people have started to obscure this musicality by eating far beyond the time the sun goes down. Those individuals who eat late around evening have demonstrated to be more helpless to stoutness and create type 2 diabetes. Discontinuous fasting permits us to complete suppers before the day and expands the period our bodies aren't getting food; this variable in your rest period where food isn't being burned-through is all considered.

Adjusting our eating routine to the circadian mood is useful for long-haul wellbeing and keeping away from illness.

Autophagy

Autophagy is intended to permit the body to throw out every one of the harmed or dead cells that the body at this point doesn't need and supplant them with more imperative, better cells that will keep on profiting the body.

Irregular fasting is enthusiastically suggested. To comprehend its elements, see it like this: when we eat, the insulin goes up, and glucagon goes down; when we don't eat, the insulin goes down, and glucagon goes up. Glucagon is a fundamental chemical in the body; the higher it is, the quicker it can invigorate autophagy from occurring inside the body.

Cell fix and recharging is the response to more slow maturing and battling sickness. The better the cells and the more cells inside our bodies, the better we are.

Keep in mind that low autophagy levels can be negative to our well-being, the same way undeniable levels can represent a danger. Therefore, there must be an even equilibrium dominated, eating and not eating, and keeping away from an existence of candidate calorie-confined eating regimens.

Improvement in Hormone Profile

There are a lot of individuals who stay away from discontinuous fasting as they feel it will cause their wellness levels to crumble. It isn't really the situation for the individuals who do partake in irregular fasting. Studies have shown that fasting doesn't adversely affect the individuals who perform standard proactive tasks, particularly if you cut down on your carbs quickly and are in a ketosis state. Studies have shown that actual preparing while at the same time fasting can prompt higher metabolic variations.

Diminishes Inflammation

Irregular fasting advances autophagy, a cycle where the body obliterates its old or harmed cells. Killing off old cells may seem like a horrendous thought. In any case, it tends to be viewed as a method of eliminating old and undesirable soil from your body. It's a basic technique for the body to clean and fix itself. Old and harmed cells can cause aggravation. Since discontinuous fasting invigorates autophagy, then, at that point, it is feasible to decrease irritation in visit b body while fasting.

Supports Healthy Bodily Functions

Discontinuous fasting gives your body time to finish cycles and capacities before bringing more food into your framework. Each time you eat, you give your body a satisfactory opportunity to use the food and use it fittingly. In current culture, we consistently gorge and push our bodies to be in a condition of processing continually. Subsequently, our frameworks become overpowered, and we don't adequately process everything. It can prompt you not to get sufficient nourishment, put away fats, and battle to create sound chemicals and synthetic substances inside your body.

Polycystic Ovarian Syndrome and Intermittent Fasting

Polycystic ovaries are a genuinely normal infection in ladies. This sickness causes a chemical move and can affect ladies' battle with weight gain and trouble getting in shape as a symptom of the infection. While there are relatively few investigations about what discontinuous fasting means for the infection, there is proof that consolidating irregular fasting with a keto diet fundamentally directed the chemicals and made weight reduction feasible for polycystic ovarian disorder patients. There is by all accounts some possible expectation with utilizing discontinuous fasting to help treat and keep up with infections like polycystic ovarian condition and other hormonal problems. Time and extra exploration will advise us if irregular fasting has a future in assisting with this infection.

Metabolic Reset

Numerous ladies, as they age, experience diminished digestion. It is mostly because of the regular maturing measure and part of the way because of harming the digestion throughout the long term. Regular accidents eating fewer carbs, helpless rest, exhaustion, chronic weakness, and more can harm your digestion, hence keeping you from getting in shape. Yet, by just rehearsing irregular fasting, you can reset and lift your digestion, permitting you to get in shape and assisting you with feeling better and keeping up with great slender muscle as you age.

Change in Cell Function

At the point when you fast for some time, various changes happen in your body. For example, your body will begin an interaction of cell fix, and there will be changes in your chemical level. A distinction in these levels makes it simpler for the body to get the put away fat. You will see a decrease in the degree of insulin, which helps increment the body's capacity to consume fat. An increment in the human development chemical assists with expanding fit muscle and consuming more fat than expected. Harmed cells are handled, and different cycles of cell fix kick in. additionally, a few changes happen inside the qualities and particles that ensure you against sickness.

Weight Reduction

The advantage of having an eating routine is weight reduction.

At the point when you follow discontinuous fasting, it will lessen the number of suppers you eat. When you eat less, the calories you devour will also diminish. When the insulin decreases, the chemical development increments alongside an increment in norepinephrine, helping the body separately and putting away fat to give energy. There is an increment in your metabolic rate when you fast—aiding the body to consume more calories. The impact of irregular fasting is two-overlap. On the opposite side, it increments and makes your body more productive while consuming fats. The decrease in the degree of food you burn diminishes your general calorie admission.

Lower the Risk of Diabetes

The most well-known medical issue that plagues humankind nowadays, aside from weight, is diabetes. High glucose prompts insulin obstruction in the body. Discontinuous fasting assists with lessening glucose and, in this manner, decreases insulin obstruction in the body. Your body can be safe, prompting an expansion in the glucose level, and the endless loop continues forever. On the off chance that you pick this eating routine, you can effectively invert this condition.

It Boosts Your Metabolic Rate

Studies show that remaining in an abstained state prompts a spike in the chemical norepinephrine. This chemical builds your basal metabolic rate and consumes fat. What's more, when you enter your eating window, your digestion actually remains at a raised level. You are almost consuming an overabundance of fat in any event when eating!

Further, Develop Muscle Health

Numerous individuals get excited about the transitory weight decrease they experience while attempting the accident diet. That is until they quit getting in shape and abandon an eating routine in the long run. Unfortunately, the majority of the weight reduction individuals accomplish on these eating regimens isn't fat misfortune but water weight and muscle weight.

Work on Mental Well Being

Poor psychological well-being is getting more normal than at any other time, with more than forty million Americans experiencing one type of dysfunctional behavior or another and numerous others battling with transient sadness and tension. Perhaps the most well-known reason for incapacity in moderately aged Americans (and the youthful individuals) is ongoing serious sorrow. However, a greater part of these individuals never looks for proficient assistance.

Cell Repair

Autophagy is the cycle of waste expulsion in the body, and discontinuous fasting helps launch this interaction. The body separates and uses broken, just as useless proteins. An expansion in autophagy shields you from a few degenerative sicknesses like disease and Alzheimer's.

This load of advantages helps to expand your life expectancy and help you have a better existence. However, you will not exclusively get thinner; however, you can likewise further develop your general well-being by following the irregular fasting strategy.

Further Developed Sex Drive

Lower levels of creation in both estrogen and testosterone may prompt a diminished sex drive. It's anything but a mental or physiological issue, yet it is a hormonal matter. Thus, when you participate in discontinuous fasting, your cerebrum will recover its equilibrium and start to deliver the right levels.

As well as working on your intellectual capacity, limiting the creation of cortisol, and boosting your state of mind through expanded creation of endorphins and dopamine, your body will likewise control the creation of estrogen and testosterone might prompt a better sex drive.

Chapter 6. Autophagy for Women Over 50

What if there is a way to stay forever young? What if you could erase a couple of years from your face and skin and take off some inches from your waistline by activating an internal cleanup process? Would you not want to know how to do that? Well, staying forever young or finding a literal fountain of youth might be unlikely. Still, you can stimulate a natural process to keep cells rejuvenated and functioning optimally for the rest of your life. That process is known as autophagy.

All about Autophagy

Reduce, reuse, and recycle is a popular phrase you're likely to hear in discussions relating to environmental sustainability. In many ways, this is similar to autophagy, which means reducing or breaking down and repairing part of the cell and then recovering important body chemicals that the liver can reuse.

In a nutshell, autophagy is the natural process that removes toxic materials and broken cells from your body to create new and healthier cells. The term comes from Latin, which translates to self-eating (auto= "self" and phagy= "to eat"). Weirdly, this means your body is eating itself! Don't panic. It's a good thing. It's a rejuvenation process for your body.

If you fully realize what autophagy is and how to make it work for you, you will be quick to find ways to consciously stimulate the process because it can keep you feeling and looking younger than your real age! Older adults, in particular, can use this natural process to increase longevity.

Here's a simple analogy of how autophagy works that I think many women can relate to. Think of what happens inside your kitchen when you are preparing a delicious meal. You are creating something heartfelt and necessary while at the same time making a mess and producing waste. If you leave your kitchen dirty after preparing your meal, it will be difficult to make your next meal. So, you do what any self-respecting woman does: throw or put away leftovers, clean the counter, put away unused ingredients, and recycle some of the food if you can. This is exactly how autophagy works in your body. It cleans up after you!

A big mess is created each day inside the body. This mess includes parts of dead cells, damaged proteins, and harmful particles that prevent optimal body function. When you were much younger, the process of autophagy cleared this mess up as quickly as possible, keeping you looking young and supple. But as you grow older, the cleanup process slows down. Dirt, mess, and crumbs start to build up internally due to old age. If left unattended, the buildup can result in rapid aging, increased risk of cancer and dementia, and other diseases associated with old age.

But growing older doesn't mean you're doomed to have an inefficient cellular cleaning process. You can stimulate the process of autophagy and make it work as it used to when you were a lot younger. An effective way to do that is by doing something that induces stress, such as decreasing insulin levels and increasing your glucagon levels. In simpler terms, go without food for longer than you usually would. When you get starving, as you do when you fast, your glucagon increases and stimulates autophagy.

You can achieve some positive life-altering benefits by simply activating autophagy. But before going into the immense health benefits, let us consider the science behind the process, albeit briefly.

The Science behind Autophagy

Autophagy in humans is induced by the activation of a protein known as p62. As soon as broken or damaged cells caused by metabolic byproducts begin to appear, p62 stimulates the process of clearing up the clutter on a cellular level. All remaining parts of waste or damaged cells that can lead to health problems are reduced, reused, and recycled. Think of the process as decluttering on a cellular level. The entire process is neatly executed to keep you healthy, strong to handle any biological stress, and keep you looking and feeling young.

Researchers from Newcastle University found that humans evolved to live longer by responding well to biological stressors (Newcastle University, 2018). Usually, fruit flies can't withstand stress. But when researchers genetically altered fruit flies by giving them the human version of p62, they found that the fruit flies lived longer than usual, even under stressful conditions.

The Benefits

Some people are said to have different biological and chronological ages. That is to say, their age is different from the quality of their life. For example, women are more likely to worry about showing signs of aging or looking older than men. Thankfully, you can look younger by activating autophagy. The process for your cells is to remove toxins and recycle cells instead of creating new ones. As a result, these rejuvenated cells will behave like new and work better.

Your skin is constantly exposed to harmful lights, air, chemicals, as well as harsh weather conditions. This causes damage to your skin cells. As the damaged cells continue to accumulate, your skin begins to wrinkle, lose elasticity, and no longer appear smooth. The process of autophagy repairs your skin cells that might have been partly damaged to make your skin glow and healthier. In the same way that wears and tear happens with things you frequently use, wear and tear (micro tear) also happens to your muscles as you use them, especially during exercises. Your muscles become inflamed and require repairs. What this means is you need more energy to use these specific muscles. The process of autophagy in your cells will degrade the damaged parts in the muscle, reduce the amount of energy sent to the muscle, and ensure energy balance.

Your cells need to be in top shape to keep your metabolism working well. The powerhouse of your cell is the mitochondria. A lot of harmful trash is left behind in the mitochondria as it performs its function of burning fat and making adenosine triphosphate (ATP). This molecule stores all the energy you need to do almost everything. This harmful trash can damage your cells. Autophagy ensures that these toxins are promptly taken care of to prevent damage to your cells and keep them in a healthy state.

During your cellular cleaning and repairs, several processes and activities also help you maintain a healthy weight. For example, when toxins are removed from your cells through autophagy, and you successfully excrete them, your fat cells can no longer store these toxins. Also, when you fast for short periods (12 to 16 hours), autophagy is activated, fat-burning also takes place, and since it is not a prolonged fast, your proteins are spared. All these activities and processes help to make you leaner and fitter.

The cells of your gastrointestinal tract hardly ever take breaks. You put them to work consistently, and this can affect digestive health. Autophagy helps repair and restore the cells. When you stop eating for long periods, you give your ample gut time to rest and heal. Giving your gut some rest (from digesting your meal) is vital for overall improved digestive health.

Chapter 7. Diet and Autophagy

Current science and research have revealed that one of the best ways to beat lifestyle ailments and complications is by taking care of the root of the illness. As you know, the body is made up of building blocks called a cell. There are trillions of cells in a person's body.

Unwanted molecules will accumulate within them over time, causing harm to some of their components. Juice cleanses and detox teas didn't equate to the body's detoxing abilities. It does this by autophagy, a normal mechanism through which the body cleans up cellular waste and maintains the processes running smoothly. According to preliminary studies, increasing autophagy will decrease inflammation, defend against disease, and help anti-aging. And if you're curious about how to trigger autophagy, there are a few options that don't need calorie restriction or the use of specific supplements.

In reality, the autophagic phase may be sped up by combining the benefits of fasting and the ketogenic diet. Intermittent fasting, exercise, and a restricted diet are one of the most effective methods to activate autophagy. Waiting only a few hours between meals, on the other hand, does not imply instant autophagy.

The body must have low liver glycogen, which involves a 14 to 16-hour fast to reach this process. The Taylor & Francis Group discovered that short-term fasting cycles of 24 hours resulted in a significant rise in the number of cells experiencing autophagy. Autophagy begins sooner, so a more practical 16:8 fast is perhaps the best place to start.

Every person is different, so this guide has put together various autophagy methods to provide alternatives and ensure that every person is covered.

What Is Autophagy?

Autophagy means "self-eating," but this is a positive thing. Your body uses autophagy to flush out dead cells and contaminants, allowing you to rebuild younger, healthier cells.

Our cells collect a mixture of dead organelles, degraded proteins, and oxidized particles over time, clogging the body's inner workings. Since cells cannot differentiate and act properly, this hastens the symptoms of aging and age-related diseases. (Autophagy should not be mistaken with apoptosis, a form of programmed cell death distinct from the clean-up of cellular degeneration.)

The importance of this lysosome-dependent cell-regeneration mechanism to your optimal health cannot be overstated. Autophagy deficiency has been attributed to several neurodegenerative diseases, including Alzheimer's disease.

Since all of our cells, such as those in the brain, would endure a lifetime, the body has evolved a special means of eliminating damaged sectors and instinctively protecting itself against disease.

How Does Autophagy Work?

Autophagy normally runs in the background, silently doing its job. It affects how the body reacts to stress, retains equilibrium, and controls cellular activity.

The cells of the body are stressed by fasting and calorie restriction. When anyone restricts the amount of food they consume, their cells receive fewer calories than they need to work properly. As a result, the cells become more efficient. Autophagy allows the body's cells to scrub out and regenerate any unused or weakened components in reaction to the stress caused by fasting or calorie restriction.

There's proof that triggering autophagy slows the aging process, reduces inflammation, and improves optimal performance. You will naturally boost your autophagy reaction to help your body avoid disease and promote longevity.

Benefits of Autophagy

While the body will clean up on its own, and autophagy is present in all cells, there are many advantages to promoting daily autophagy:

- Protects the nervous and immune systems by regulating cellular mitochondria, which increases energy output in the body.
- Helps to prevent metabolic stress.
- Enhances cognitive capacity and protects against cardiac disease by encouraging new cells' growth, especially in the brain and heart tissue.
- Aids in the maintenance and restoration of the intestinal lining, which helps to enhance digestive efficiency.
- Maintains the purity and durability of our DNA, which helps to preserve our genomes.

- Genetic connections between autophagy deficiencies and cancer have been identified, adding to the growing body of evidence that autophagy is a genuine tumor suppressor pathway.

Ways to Induce Autophagy to Keep Your Cells Fresh

You can speed up the body's autophagy process in a variety of ways. These five basic measures increase the autophagy mechanism to cleanse your cells, reduce inflammation, and keep the body functioning smoothly. Remember that autophagy is a stress reaction, so you'll have to trick your body into believing it's under siege. Here's how to do it:

1. Eat a High-Fat, Low-Carb Diet

Since fat differs from protein, it must be the most important macronutrient in our diets. Protein will transform into a carb and sugar, but fat cannot. A keto diet, in particular, offers you an advantage when it comes to autophagy. The switch from burning glucose (carbs) to ketones (fats) mimics what happens in the body when it is fasted, which may improve autophagy in and of itself.

2. Go on a Protein Fast

Limit your protein intake to 15g-25g a day once or twice a week. This allows the body to recycle proteins for an entire day, which helps relieve stress and cleanse your cells without causing muscle loss. During this time, the body is compelled to eat its proteins and contaminants rather than incoming amino acids since autophagy is triggered.

3. Practice Intermittent Fasting

According to research, autophagy and fasting can go hand in hand since you can speed up the autophagic process by restricting the eating window. Intermittent fasting is linked to weight loss, improved insulin sensitivity, and a lower risk of disease.

4. Exercise

Another reason to join the gym. Exercise has been found to assist autophagy activation; all training methods promote autophagy, supporting the notion that all movement is good movement.

High-intensity interval training is more recommended, and for autophagy, the "less is more" strategy to exercise is emphasized. The easiest approach to enabling autophagy is to do 30 minutes of weightlifting and strength training workouts every day. Since autophagy thrives on the stress of interval training, it's just about bringing in short-term, intense stress.

5. Get Restorative Sleep

According to researchers, you will benefit from autophagy even though you're sleeping. Autophagy seems to imitate circadian patterns, according to a 2016 rat report, and sleep fragmentation or brief sleep interruptions seem to disturb autophagy.

How to Induce Autophagy with Intermittent Fasting

Intermittent fasting is one of the simplest ways to begin a healthy and successful fasting practice that has been shown to upregulate or improve autophagy. The alternating method between times of free feeding and periods of limited eating is known as intermittent fasting. Instead of actively grazing, the body can cause autophagy and bring cellular clean-up to function by making this strong distinction between eating and not eating. Autophagy is activated while you are fasting or not feeding.

Autophagy is most likely to account for Intermittent fasting health advantages. As you fast, your insulin levels decrease, which stimulates autophagy. When you eat, insulin levels rise, and autophagy gets blocked. Insulin assists in the transfer of sugar (glucose) through cells from the bloodstream; in addition to fasting, a low carb or keto diet is also helpful for autophagy.

16:8 is the most popular form of intermittent fasting. This is where you limit your diet and fast for 16 hours before resuming normal eating for 8 hours. Some people prefer 18:6 because of the additional two hours of autophagy advantages.

In several aspects, practicing intermittent fasting autophagy will help you achieve fantastic outcomes in your quest to enhance your fitness. By combining these important resources, you will enable the body to function at its highest on a deep cellular level.

Alternate your intermittent fasting schedule if you want a longer or shorter intermittent fasting time.

Chapter 8. Metabolic Autophagy Foods

Food That Boosts the Autophagy Process

The amount of exercise needed for switching on the autophagy boost is hard to find out.

1. Clean Water

Even though you aren't eating, it's crucial for so many reasons to stay hydrated for the health of basically every critical organ in your body. The amount of water every person should drink varies, but at all times, you want your urine to be a pale-yellow color. Dark yellow urine shows fatigue that can lead to headaches, tiredness, and light-headedness. Combined with little food, it may be a disaster recipe. If you are not excited by the prospect of plain water, add a squeeze of lemon juice, cucumber slices, or a few mint leaves to your tea. It is going to be our little secret.

2. Avocado

Consuming the most potent calorie fruit when striving to lose weight may sound counterintuitive.

3. Catch

There is a justification for eating at least eight ounces of fish per week in the Dietary Guidelines. It is rich in healthy fats and protein and contains sufficient amounts of vitamin D. If you eat only a limited amount of food throughout the day, don't you want one that provides your buck with more nutrient bang? It might mess with your cognition to limit your calorie intake, and fish is often considered a "brain food."

4. Cruciferous Vegetables

Foods like broccoli, sprouts from Brussels, and cauliflower are all packed with the f-word — fiber. Eating fiber-rich foods that will keep you regular and prevent constipation is crucial when you are eating erratically. Fiber also has the potential to make you feel complete, which is something you would want if you don't have 16 hours to eat again.

5. Cocktails

I was hoping you could repeat after me: The white foods are not all bad. Another study found potato eating as part of a healthy diet might help with weight loss. Sorry, not counting French fries and potato chips.

5. Legumes and Beans

Your favorite addition to chili on the IF lifestyle might be your best friend. Food, mainly carbs, provides energy for activity. Although we're not telling you to carbo-load, tossing some low-calorie carbohydrates, such as beans and legumes, into your eating plan would certainly not hurt. Besides, foods such as chickpeas, black beans, peas, and lentils have been shown to decrease body weight, even without limited calories.

6. Antibiotics

Do you know what you like most about the little bitters in your gut? Diversity and continuity. That means, that when they are hungry, they are not happy. And you may experience some irritating side effects, like constipation, when your gut is not happy. To counteract this unpleasantness, add foods that are rich in probiotics to your diet, such as kefir, kombucha, or kraut. The Farmhouse Culture Gut Shots are great for any 500 calorie day, as every 1.5-ounce shot is full of live probiotics (10 billion CFUs) for only ten calories.

7. Berry

Your favorite addition to the smoothie is packed with essential nutrients. And that's not even the best part — a new study showed that people who ate a flavonoid-rich diet, including those in blueberries and strawberries, had smaller rises in BMI over 14 years than those who didn't eat berries.

8. Eggs Proceed

One large egg is filled with six grams of protein and cooks for minutes. Getting as much protein as possible is crucial to keep your muscles full and build up. In other words, why not hard-boil some eggs when you are looking for something to do during your fasting period?

9. Muzzles

They may be higher in calories than most snacks, but there is something in nuts that most junk food doesn't contain — good fat. Work indicates that polyunsaturated fat in walnuts may also change the hunger and satiety physiological markers.

And if you think about calories, then don't! Research conducted in 2012 showed that a one-ounce serving of almonds (about 23 nuts) had 20 percent fewer calories than those on the bottle.

10. Full Grains

It seems like being on a diet and eating carbs belong in two different buckets, but it is not always like that! Plus, a new study suggests consuming whole grains rather than refined grains could potentially revive your metabolism. So go ahead and eat all your grains, and try faro, bulgur, spelt, Kamut, amaranth, millet, sorghum, or freekeh out of your comfort zone.

Chapter 9. Get Started/How to Plan?

Intermittent fasting is one of the easiest lifestyles to follow. It has immense health benefits. The majority of people believe that in order for anything to succeed, it must be complicated. For intermittent fasting, this is not the case.

Maintaining strict eating and fasting windows is at the core of intermittent fasting.

Eating Window

First, let us begin with the easier part. This is the window in which you are allowed to eat.

This book is especially for women over 50, but let us first talk about women in general. Food is very important for the hormonal balance of women. Prolonged food deprivation can cause hormonal imbalance. This is why women of their reproductive age are advised against strict calorie-restrictive diets or even fasting for very long periods.

Studies conducted on mice demonstrate that longer food deprivation of any kind for a consistent period can cause shrinkage in the reproductive organs. It can also affect hormonal secretion.

Therefore, young women should only practice only moderate intermittent fasting. Their fasts should not be longer than 14 hours. They should not even start with 14-hour fasts, to begin with. They should help their bodies adapt to the change slowly and gradually.

When it comes to women over 50, longer fasts can be performed without restrictions. The risk of hormonal imbalances causing irregular periods or complications in conception and childbearing is not there.

Women over 50 have greater freedom in terms of the duration of fasts they want to undertake. This presents a very advantageous opportunity.

Women have a greater affinity to accumulate fat, but they are also more likely to shed the fat fast under the right conditions. Longer fasts help begin the process of ketosis, and hence, women can lose weight and burn fat much faster than men.

Hence, the hormonal conundrum that is a great problem for younger women doesn't challenge women over 50.

Women over 50 reaching their menopause get freedom from issues like menstruation. While this may be a great relief, other issues become more prominent.

For instance, problems like PCOS start troubling more where they should also have gone with their reproductive abilities. However, this doesn't happen.

Intermittent fasting with a correct diet can also help you manage PCOS symptoms to a great extent. Frequent chills, mood swings, obesity, glucose tolerance issues, and other problems will not arise if you practice intermittent fasting.

Getting back to eating, women over 50 can take the liberty of holding longer fasts safely as they get more accustomed to fasting. They are at a lower risk of health issues arising due to hormonal imbalances caused by food deprivation.

Eating Hours in the Fasting Window

While women younger than 50 are not advised to fast for longer than 14–16 hours, if you have crossed your 50s, you can safely take it a notch higher to 18 or even 20 hours if you feel like it.

However, in intermittent fasting, the number of calories you can eat holds very little importance, and the way and hours within which you eat them are way more important.

This means that your whole eating window, which spans from the time of the beginning of your fast until you finish the last meal of the day, is very important. This period is the eating window.

If you begin your breakfast at 7 in the morning and finish your last meal of the day by 5 in the evening, then you will have a 10-hour window.

Eating Discipline—Culling the Habit of Snacking

Another essential part of the eating window is following an eating discipline. You will have to improve your habit of eating.

We all eat mindlessly. We eat for the sake of eating. We don't mind having a few bites when invited to eat, although we may not have any appetite or hunger.

We feel it comfortably fine to have a glass of cold drink when offered by someone even when we are not hungry, not realizing the fact that the glass of soft drink may have an equal number of calories as a full meal. To top it all, they are empty calories which are even more dangerous.

We get tempted to eat when an intoxicating aroma of food passes through our nostrils. Likewise, our desire to eat goes up when we see sweets and desserts on display.

We like to eat when we are sad as there are foods that provide great comfort. It is a sad fact that there is a category of food categorized as comfort food in restaurants.

We may only have two proper meals or less in 1 day but may have up to 10 incidents on average that may cause insulin spikes.

This is the habit of snacking that is causing the highest amount of damage to our system. Our digestive system gets crushed under a load of food, and it is unable to process that much food. This leads to the passing of most nutrients through the stool unabsorbed.

It also causes irreparable damage to our insulin system, causing insulin resistance. It overloads your whole pancreatic system making it overwork, and the beta cells may lose the ability to produce the required amount of insulin in the future; this problem is known as diabetes.

The most important step toward following eating discipline is to stop eating indiscriminately. You will have to put an end to the habit of snacking. This is a habit that is only taking you towards a health doom.

You can only have 2–3 nutrient-dense meals in a day that can help in providing nutrition and energy.

Too many women fail at this; this can sound intimidating, but it comes very naturally with practice.

You will have to begin by lowering the number of snacks you have in a day and then bring it to a minimum.

You will also have to eliminate sweets and refined carbs from your diet as they lead to food cravings. The sweeter you will have your diet, the faster you will feel more inclined to eat. If you have more fat and protein in your diet, you will feel less inclined to eat as your gut takes much longer to process them, and they keep releasing energy at a steady rate for much longer.

This is the basic preparation before you begin intermittent fasting. You must remember that intermittent fasting is not some magical formula; it is a way to discipline the body to perform in an ideal way. This can't happen if you practice intermittent fasting but don't stop having snacks at short intervals in your eating windows. This would keep causing insulin spikes, and your system would remain under duress.

Another thing with snacks is that they are mostly made up of refined flour and sweets. This makes them addictive, and you have stronger cravings for them. There are no snacks rich in fat and protein as they would become proper meals then, and you are less likely to feel inclined to eat after having them.

Therefore, eliminate snacks from your life, and you will be able to get the benefits of intermittent fasting.

Fasting Window

Fasting windows are much simpler. There are very few restrictions in place apart from the eating ban. You can't eat in your fasting window is a comprehensive term, and it also includes the consumption of calories even through drinking.

You are allowed to drink water, and it is very helpful to drink plenty of water as and when you feel thirsty. This will help your body in flushing out the toxins during the initial cleaning phase. But besides water, there are very few things that you can safely consume.

You can't drink any kind of sweetened beverage. You can't consume anything that has calories, even a few. This leaves out all kinds of sweetened soft drinks, alcoholic beverages, fruits, and other such things. There needs to be a complete blanket ban on the consumption of calories in any form.

For women, in general, the fasting windows can range anywhere from 14–16 hours. However, if you are a woman over 50 and have been practicing intermittent fasting for quite some time, you can experiment with longer fasts as long as you feel comfortable.

There is only one simple rule when you get accustomed to longer fasts: not to overdo things. Try to maintain a routine.

Routine

It is a very important topic that seldom gets any limelight in weight loss, but it is equally important, like everything else. If you don't follow a routine, you will find it increasingly difficult to follow a fasting schedule.

Have you ever noticed that some people eat very less or after very long intervals, and they don't feel hungry, while you may find it hard to stay away from food even for short intervals?

This happens because our hunger system works like clockwork.

Another interesting fact is that hunger pangs are temporary. This means that if you stop paying attention to these hunger pangs and divert your attention to something else, you may not feel the hunger pangs after some time. Again, this happens because the ghrelin release is limited.

This is important to understand because shifting your fasting timings can have a toll on your tolerance.

For instance, if you start beginning your fasts around 6 in the evening and break your fasts at 10 in the morning, your ghrelin release would get timed accordingly after a few days. This means that you will start having strong hunger pangs in the morning at around 10 and around 6 in the evening to facilitate the intake of food. This would also mean that you will feel less inclined to eat during your fasting window.

However, if you follow an erratic fasting routine in which you begin your fast one day at 4 in the evening, 6 on another day, and at 8 on yet another day, your ghrelin release would never be able to time itself, and you will have to see longer periods of hunger pangs.

You will have frequent gastric juice released in your system when there is no food to digest, and that can also cause problems like flatulence and acid reflux.

Therefore, it is crucial that you follow a fixed routine in your fasting schedule and don't change the timings very often. This will help you in practicing fasting in a much easier way.

Chapter 10. How to Write Down Your Goals

A goal is a mental representation of a specific and measurable result that you want to reach through a commitment to specific actions. There may be a dream or hope at its base, but a goal is quantifiable, unlike dreams. With a well-written goal, you will know what you want to get and how you intend to get it. Writing personal goals can be both incredibly satisfying and widely useful. Some studies have shown that setting goals for your intermittent fasting protocol can help you feel much safer and more confident, even when it comes to long-term fasting periods. As the Chinese philosopher Lao Tzu said: "A thousand miles trip starts with a single step." You can start taking the journey that will take you to the desired destination by writing down your personal weight loss goals.

Reflect on What Is Considered Significant

Studies show that when your goals concern something that you consider motivating, you are more likely to reach them. Next, identify the areas of your life in which you would like to make changes. It is normal for every area to have rather large borders in this initial phase. Generally, people decide to give themselves goals in terms of self-improvement and physical health. An accurate intermittent fasting protocol can help you move toward these two directions at the same time.

You should start by drafting out your goals on a piece of paper. For example, you may want to make significant changes in health and physical well-being areas. Write down this information, specifying what you would like to change.

At this stage, you could indicate the goals in vague terms. It is normal. As for health, for example, you could write "improve physical form" or "healthy eating."

Identify Your "Best Self"

Studies suggest that determining which you think is the best possible version of yourself can help you feel more positive and satisfied with your life. No less important, it is a way to understand the goals you really consider significant. Identifying what is the "best yourself as possible" requires two steps. First of all, you have to see yourself in the future once you reach your goals and evaluate the qualities you need to get to that point.

Imagine a moment in the future when you have become the best possible version of yourself. How will you be? What things will you give more importance to? At this point, it is essential to concentrate on what "yourself" considers important, ignoring the pressures and desires of others.

Imagine the details of this "future you" and think positive. You can think about something that is the "dream of your life," a fundamental stage of your weight loss journey, or some other significant result. For example, your best self could be a healthy woman who easily follows an intermittent fasting protocol. In this case, imagine what you would do. Which intermittent fasting protocol would you follow? How many calories would you eat per day?

Please, put as many details of your best self when writing down your goals. Imagine what qualities your "best self" is using to achieve success. For example, assuming that you follow an intermittent fasting protocol, you would surely know how to meal prep and manage hunger. Those are two skills you just discovered you must develop to improve your health.

Once you have a list of the skills you need to develop, think about which of these qualities you already have. Be honest with yourself, not severe. Then reflect on the qualities you can develop. Imagine ways to be able to develop the habits and skills you need. For example, if you want to follow an intermittent fasting protocol but you have no knowledge about eating healthy, you can buy a few books about this topic. The beauty of knowledge is that it can be acquired.

Fix Priorities for Different Areas

Once you have filled out a list of areas in which you would like to make changes, you have to put them in order of priority. Trying to improve all aspects of your life at once is likely to end up with you feeling exhausted, running the risk of failing to achieve your goals because they seem impossible.

Divide your goals into three distinct units:

- General goals
- Second-level goals
- Third-level goals

The first is the most important because they are the ones who feel more significant to you. Those of the second and third levels are relevant, but you do not give them the same value as the general goals. They also tend to be more specific.

An example might be helpful. At the general level, you might want to "give priority to your health by following an intermittent fasting protocol." You may want to "be a good friend, keep the house clean, and be a good parent at the second level." You might want to "Learn to knit or become more efficient at work at the third level."

Start Narrowing the Field

When you have established the areas you would like to change, and what changes you would like to make, you can start determining the specifications of what you would like to achieve. These specifications will be the basis of your goals. By answering some questions, you will be able to identify the who, the what, the when, the where, and the results you want to achieve.

Studies carried out suggest that formulating a specific goal increases the chances of being able to reach it and helps you feel happier about the changes it requires.

Determine the Who

When you formulate a goal, it is important to determine who is responsible for achieving every sub-goal. Since we are talking about personal goals, the responsible likely is you. Nevertheless, some goals require the cooperation of others, so it is useful to identify who will be responsible for those parts.

For example, "following an intermittent fasting protocol" is a personal goal that probably only involves you. Otherwise, if your goal is "helping my entire family follow an intermittent fasting protocol," it will also be necessary to contemplate the responsibility of other people.

Determine the What

Asking yourself this question helps you define the goal and the details and results you want. For example, "following an intermittent fasting protocol" is a goal too wide to be manageable. It lacks precision. Reflect on the details of what you want to learn to do. "Follow an intermittent fasting protocol and lose 10lbs in 5 weeks" is more specific.

The more details you can add to the what, the clearer the steps you will have to take to achieve your goal.

Determine the When

One of the key factors in correctly formulating your goals is to divide them into different stages. Knowing when you have to reach every specific step can help you stay on the right track while giving you a clear feeling of progressing.

Be realistic in setting the different stages you want to reach. "Losing five pounds by following an intermittent fasting protocol" is not something that can occur from one week to another. Reflect on how long it is really necessary to reach every stage of your plan.

Determine the Were

It may be useful to identify a certain place where you will reach your goal in many cases. For example, if what you are pursuing is following an intermittent fasting protocol three times a week, it is good to decide if you intend to cook at home, buy food on the go or have it delivered to your house. It might seem useless to write down so many details, but trust us when we say that they can make or break your ability to achieve your goals.

Determine the How

This step urges you to imagine how you intend to reach every stage of the process to achieve your goal. This way, you will define the structure more precisely, and you will have a clear idea of the actions you have to do to complete each phase.

Returning to the intermittent fasting protocol example, you will need to choose a meal plan, get the ingredients, have the necessary tools, and find the time to prepare your meals in the kitchen.

Determine the Why

As mentioned above, the chances of being able to achieve your goal increase proportionately to how significant and motivating it feels. Determining the reason behind your goal helps you understand the motivation that drives you to achieve a certain goal.

In our example, you may want to follow an intermittent fasting protocol to feel more attractive and be healthy.

It is important to keep the "why" in mind while you do the actions necessary to achieve your goals. Giving you highly specific goals is useful, but you also need always to have a clear motivation that pushes you when things get difficult.

Write Your Goals in Positive Terms

Research shows that you are more likely to reach your goals if you express them in positive terms. In other words, write them considering them something towards which you are moving, not something you want to avoid.

For example, if one of your goals is to follow an intermittent fasting protocol, a motivating way to express it would be: "eat only from 6 pm to midnight."

On the contrary, "not eat from midnight to 6 pm" is not very encouraging or motivating. Words become things, so be careful in what words you decide to use.

Make Sure Your Goals Are Based on Performance

Succeeding certainly requires hard work and strong motivation, but you must also be sure of setting goals that your commitment allows you to reach. You can control only your actions, not those of others and not the results.

Focus your goals on the actions you can do yourself instead of specific results. By conceiving success as a performance process, you will be able to feel that you have remained faithful to the commitment made even on the occasions when the result is not the one you hoped.

Define Your Strategy

These are the actions and tactics you intend to use to achieve your goals. Break down the strategy into individual concrete tasks as it makes it even easier to put yourself into practice. Furthermore, it helps you monitor progress. Use the answers you gave to the preceding questions (what, where, when, etc.) to determine your strategy.

Determine the Time Frame

For example, "following an intermittent fasting protocol for a day" is something you can start doing immediately. Instead, you will have to sustain a much longer effort for other goals.

Divide Your Plan into Individual Tasks

Once you have determined the destination, you need to reach, and at what time you have to do it, you can divide your strategy into smaller and concrete tasks. In practice, you can determine the individual actions you have to do to reach that goal. Give yourself a deadline for each of them to know if you respect your plans.

Chapter 11. Exercises to Do During Intermittent Fasting for Women Over 50

Physical activity is the last piece of the weight loss triad, but it is not less important. Exercising increases blood flow, activates endorphins after and during workouts and can aid in calorie burn. The amount of calories you burn is determined by the exercise's form, length, and strength. However, this is generally a small amount and is nowhere near the number of calories you burn from the basal metabolic rate. The average Joe will not have the time or resources to devote significant attention to burning calories. Instead, exercise helps in other ways. Intermittent fasting, for example, will help control your energy levels by depleting available glycogen reserves, causing your body to burn fat if it isn't already doing so. Remember those old-school workout videos with everyone talking about "feeling the burn?" Very rarely will exercise directly burn fat. In fact, fat only gets burned after glycogen stores are gone (which takes a while). Most amateur athletes never get to that level of performance. We sometimes hear that burning x amounts of calories (3,500, for example) equals burning 1 pound of fat. More specifically, you are burning 3,500 calories, which results in losing one pound of fat, more or less.

Many people feel that exercising on an empty stomach is bad. This could be true by causing a significant drop in blood sugar levels. Here, people with diabetes need to be extra careful. The best time for them to exercise would be just hours after starting a fast—when food energy is still running high in the body. An exercise of any kind will naturally bring blood sugar levels down. If someone can't regulate blood sugar levels efficiently (diabetes), they risk having a serious episode of low blood sugar. Otherwise, the body can detect that blood sugar levels are dropping and make an adequate response to metabolize glycogen. People who find it difficult to exercise while fasting may elect to "cheat" by having a small meal before the workout. Protein shakes are notorious for this, as they tend to be high in both carbohydrates and proteins. Depending on how much powder is used, mixing whey protein with water may run anywhere between 120 and 400 calories. Mixing it with milk will increase the calorie content significantly. But normally, protein shakes aren't required to get through exercise.

If you are already acclimatized to the fat-burning stage of a low-carb diet, you will find it easier to get through regular exercise, even when fasting. Trying to get a full workout in during the first week of Keto will prove difficult. Trying to exercise in the middle of a fast is also hard because you will suffer from the symptoms of low blood sugar. Diabetics will need to take precautions against them. Since a diabetic should be monitoring blood sugar levels regularly, they should schedule a blood meter test shortly before deciding to exercise. If their blood sugar is too low, they simply shouldn't do the workout. At the very least, they should eat something to get these levels back to a range that is healthy for physical activity. As with fasting, the workout should be terminated if you experience any symptoms of increased dizziness, lightheadedness, vomiting, or loss of consciousness.

The types of exercise you decide on undertaking will depend on your fitness goals. A good general recommendation for people who wish to be healthier is resistance training at least twice a week alongside the recommended 150 minutes a week of moderate to intense aerobic activity. These 150 minutes can further be increased to 300 minutes to receive even more benefits. These include lowering the risk of cardiovascular disease, reducing the risk of cancers, and a greater increase in weight-loss potential from physical activity alone. Whether a full 300 minutes of exercise is sustainable a week while fasting will depend on the person's fitness level and the fasting routine—for example, somebody who is doing the "5:2" Method may simply decide not to exercise on their fasting days, others who fast daily by skipping breakfast (and fasting overnight) may decide to get the workout done after the fasting period is over. Breaking the fast with a small meal and then doing the workout afterwards is a good option. Exercise gets a little trickier on those longer (1–3 days or more) fasts. However, the considerations are still the same, and the risk of a low blood sugar episode increases.

Benefits of Exercising While Fasted

While you can expect working out on an empty stomach to be a challenge, there are many benefits. First, working out with no food in your system means that calories expended directly take a hit on your glycogen stores. In the short term, this means that you will lose weight quickly from the water stored in glycogen and may accelerate fat burning. Along with burning the glycogen, you can expect cellular processes to burn at least some fat. There are called AMP kinases and are responsible for jump-starting fat metabolism in muscles during workouts. They only burn fat when the body detects that there isn't enough caloric energy to go around from glucose. The real nitty-gritty of what happens during exercise while fasted can get complicated fast, but your body secretes all sorts of things. Muscles that are exposed to undue oxidative stress from exercising while fasting becomes resilient to such stress over time, preventing the pace of the aging process. The brain and muscle tissues enter a rejuvenation process similar to autophagy that keeps things running smoothly. These effects are mostly stimulated during short, intense workouts like HIT workouts and resistance training.

Small amounts of human growth hormone (HGH) are also released if you exercise when glucose stores are low. In turn, this stimulates the secretion of androgens like testosterone that fuel libido and increase lean muscle mass.

Aerobic Exercise

Anything that gets you on your feet and moving around is considered aerobic. In specific, it deals with raising your heart rate for extended periods. It comes from the word that means "with oxygen," causing you to breathe faster than usual while giving your body enough oxygen to flow in the blood. Walking, jogging, jump rope, cycling, stair climbing, and countless sports all qualify for aerobic exercise. Current American physical activity guidelines recommend at least 150 minutes of this type of exercise a week. One of the most common activities you can do is walking. Walking is almost always free and can provide a welcome change of scenery. You can take your dog or a buddy along with you to keep you company.

Aerobic exercise while fasted will use glycogen primarily as fuel, depending on how far into the fast you are. If you exercise just after your last meal, you can get an energy boost from that. Believe it or not, people who work out during their fasting period report higher energy levels than they do during non-fasted workouts. This has primarily to do with the body's secretion of HGH, among other things, to compensate for the lack of readily available energy. But these levels of energy are usually reserved for people who are used to fasting. If you try to exercise during your first weeks of trying it out, expect major resistance from your body. It is prudent to take things slow and gradually increase the intensity or duration of fasted workouts. In the meantime, you can exercise on non-fasting days as usual.

Anaerobic Exercise

The opposite of aerobic exercise is the anaerobic kind. This covers different forms of resistance training, including bodyweight exercises, strength conditioning, and weight lifting. Also covered here are high-intensity workouts like HIT and sprint training. In general, anaerobic exercise and resistance training are good for creating muscle and strengthening bones. The nervous system also benefits from the mind-body connection used with resistance training. Resistance is effectively teaching the muscles how to interface with signals from the brain. Both anaerobic and aerobic exercise should be used together to get maximum weight loss results.

The key difference is that the oxygen that reaches the body through the lungs is insufficient to keep the exercise going under anaerobic conditions. Instead, muscles need to break down sugars (glycogen) to get their energy. This breakdown facilitates weight loss by reducing the amount of available glycogen at a given time. Broken down glycogen stores are converted into lactic acid buildup, which is why muscles feel sore following an intense workout.

The breakdown of muscles also elicits a repair mechanism to mend torn muscle fibers and flush out dead components from cells. You should instantly recognize this as autophagy. You will experience a boost in metabolism that lasts hours after your workout, whether you are in a fasting state or not.

Working with the Fast, Not Against It

The base rule for working out while fasting is not to push things. If you at any time feel dizzy, get migraines, start vomiting, etc., in the middle of the workout, it is not a challenge to push yourself forward, but it is a sign that you need to stop. This is especially true if you are exercising in a hot climate, as the temperature will cause your body to work overtime to keep you cool.

Hydration is important, as dehydration is a leading cause of heatstroke. If you plan on lifting heavy weights for anaerobic exercise, make sure you work with a lighter weight than usual during fasting days. Lifting heavy with insufficient glycogen stores is a good way to pass out in front of everyone at the gym. Not fun.

Chapter 12. Tricks to Get the Best Start on Intermittent Fasting for Women Over 50

Keep Your Mind Busy

It is possible to break all your barriers with the help of this. Whenever you have no work to do or feel bored, you will tend to search for some food items or snacks for munching. Boredom is the evilest thing that can gradually creep into your mind. It can make you destroy your fasting routine. You might end up having something that is not recommended for your diet and health. While watching movies, we all love to munch on something. What is the reason behind this? The answer is dopamine. It is the hormone that makes us feel happy when we provide ourselves with something that we want.

The happy feeling that you get after munching on your favorite snack doesn't only happen to you. It works for all. Dopamine can make the journey of fasting feel very hard. What is the solution to such a problem? First, you will have to keep your mind distracted by something. Try to stay busy with something that doesn't have any kind of connection with food. Next time when you feel like snacking in the middle of your fasting window, try to distract yourself. You can make yourself busy with some work or watch something interesting on the TV. The primary aim is to shift your focus.

Hydrate Yourself

You might stop yourself from having water or beverages like tea or coffee during fasting. But it is also important to keep yourself hydrated all the time. You can set reminders at different times of the day, especially during the window of fasting to hydrate yourself. Try to have a minimum of 2–3 liters of water every day. It can help you to stay full while keeping you hydrated.

Opt for Fast after Dinner

Opting for fasting right after dinner is often considered the most useful among the several intermittent fasting types. When you start with your fast after having your dinner, you will be spending most of the time in bed, sleeping. If you opt for the 16:8 method, you can read a book or watch TV for 3 hours before you sleep. Then, you will get the chance to fast continuously for 12 hours without any obstruction. So, starting with the 16:8 method is often considered the easiest type of fasting. With the help of this advice, you will be able to bring about some serious changes in your lifestyle. You will gain more control over your hunger and cravings. You can concentrate on losing weight without any need to think about what to eat.

Break the Fast Steadily and Slowly

After successfully spending many hours without any food, you might think of yourself as a human vacuum that can suck up everything on the plate. However, gulping your food in no time will be of no help to your body. You will need to chew your food properly and eat slowly. You will need to allow the system digestion to process the food fully. In this way, you can better understand your fullness so that you can prevent yourself from overeating.

Maintain Balanced Meals

Having a proper mixture of fiber, carbs, healthy fats, and protein can help shed the extra pounds and fight extreme hunger while fasting. An example of a balanced meal is grilled chicken with mashed potato and sautéed veggies with olive oil and garlic. If you want to include fruits in your meals, opt for the ones that come with a low glycemic index. Choose those fruits which are digested, metabolized, and absorbed slowly. It can help in raising blood glucose slowly. When you have a stable level of blood sugar, you can easily avoid all your cravings. Thus, having a balanced meal is the key to shedding extra pounds successfully.

Avoid Overeating

Only because you are out of the fasting window doesn't mean you can have a feast. Eating excessively will make you feel uncomfortable and bloated, but it can also destroy your weight loss goals. Overeating can have adverse effects on intermittent fasting. It doesn't matter how much food you have on your plate during the eating window. What is presented on your plate is all that matters.

Experiment with Time Periods

You can always pay attention to your lifestyle to find out which fasting method suits you the best. For instance, if you wake up early in the morning, you can have your meals in the earlier hours, like 09:00 A.M. to 05:00 P.M. You can then continue with the fast till 09:00 A.M. the next day. The real beauty of intermittent fasting lies in its flexibility. Another great option is to cut yourself off from eating earlier and then have your breakfast the next day. Human beings generally fast daily as we sleep at night. So, you can try to wrap up all your meals by 09:00 P.M. and then don't have anything until 08:00 A.M. the next morning. That is already a natural fast for 11 hours! You can extend this time slowly for long periods of fasting.

Opt for Satiating Meals

After you start with the fasting process, you will need to have satiating meals. If you fail to do so, you might start feeling demotivated, regardless of your efforts to stay within the fasting routine. Most people lose their motivation to stick to intermittent fasting because of this reason. You will need to make a concise effort to maintain the regime of fasting. You can fix a normal diet in this way:

- A simple egg recipe at breakfast.
- A simple chicken or egg recipe with some veggies for lunch.
- Having some protein supplements after exercising.
- Something bland again for dinner.

If you have some excess time left in your daily routine, you can have some nuts and fruits for snacks. Such a type of diet will surely end with dissatisfaction. You might also feel the urge to quit the practice. You might also have the worst cravings with a diet of this kind. So, what is the solution?

- Try to exclude breakfast from your meal routine. Have some coffee or water that comes with a low-calorie count.
- For your lunch, you can have the same fish or chicken meal. But try to pair it with something interesting. You can add some BBQ seasoning for extra flavor and taste.
- Consume some protein supplements after finishing your workout.
- If you want to have your dinner, you can repeat the same meal as your lunch. However, ensure you don't opt for processed food items.

In this way, you will be able to maintain your interest in the process of intermittent fasting.

Adapt Your Exercise Routine

Indeed, you can exercise while fasting. But you are required to be mindful of the types of movements that you decide to do. Also, the time when you decide to exercise plays an important role. If you want to exercise in your fasting window, try to complete your workout as soon as you get up. It will provide you with the majority of the energy. If you are not fueling the body muscles adequately, the chances of injury are high. So, choosing low-impact exercises, like cardio or yoga, is always suggested for fasting mornings. Then, you can complete your hardcore exercise session during the latter half of the day after you have your meals.

Keep Track of the Journey

Whether you believe it or not, keeping a food journal can help in maintaining a fasting diet. As you keep a note of your emotions, hunger level, weaknesses, cravings, etc., while fasting, you can gauge your progress in a better way. You can also come across some of the trigger points that might make your practice fasting harder for you.

Start Listening to the Body

It is important. Try to keep an eye on all your symptoms like fatigue, dizziness, headache, irritability, difficulty focusing, and anxiety. If you are experiencing any of these, listening to your body and breaking the fast is recommended. These are the signs that indicate your body is slowly getting into the mode of starvation.

No matter which method you choose, be patient. Your body will take some time to get accustomed to the fasting routine. Feeling hungry and weak are normal as you start fasting. So, there is no need to flip out. However, if such challenges persist for a long time, you must ditch the practice. Search for something else to meet all your goals.

Chapter 13. Other Tips to Follow to Make It More Effective

Find a Worthy Goal

First things first: find a goal that is worth pursuing, or else you will drop the idea at the first sign of resistance. If you don't have a goal that represents a strong ideal, it won't be long before you start telling yourself, "I think I've passed the stage of such childishness." And yes, many women start a new lifestyle change for reasons that they can't keep up when things get tough. For example, the desire to look like models on TV or on social media makes losing weight feel socially acceptable and ok to keep up with trends that can be harmful. Unfortunately, these reasons are not enough to keep anyone committed to a full lifestyle change, and few wonder why so many people with goals are quick to jump from one lifestyle to another.

Don't go into fasting intermittently because it is the thing to do at the moment. Instead, look for inspiring goals such as:

- Staying fit, young, and healthy.
- Improving your cognitive or brain functions.
- Improving your overall vitality and increasing energy levels.
- Balancing hormones, especially during menopausal or post-menopausal stages of life.
- Improving your overall health, thereby increasing longevity.

Surely at this stage of your life, you are aware of the inherent risks of doing something merely because others are doing it too. That type of motivation will fail you.

Check Your Hormones

A woman's hormones can be easily thrown out of whack by the slightest change in her already established pattern of behavior. Whether it is a physical change such as altering you're eating pattern or an emotional change such as being irritated or sad, it can bring about hormonal imbalance in a woman, even if it is temporary.

But for premenopausal and menopausal women, hormones can go haywire for reasons even they can't define. She could be feeling really great all week, and without anything changing, she could suddenly become fatigued, depressed, and not in the right frame of mind. These changes happen due to the unpredictability of this phase of a woman's life. Because this can happen for no apparent reason, it is best to check your hormonal levels before putting your body through a major lifestyle change. If you've ever had thyroid, cortisol, or adrenal fatigue issues, ensure that you have these checks before you begin.

So, as you grow older and begin to experience a decline in your estrogen and progesterone levels, your testosterone levels are also taking a nosedive. Your libido can be affected by low testosterone levels and make you feel exhausted and bummed out for no reason at all. So while you are checking your other hormones, don't forget to do a testosterone test. The thyroid and testosterone hormones also help in weight regulation. So, if you intend to shed some weight using intermittent fasting, these tests are very necessary.

Start Slow

To go from having five or six meals daily to eating only once a day can lead to very dire consequences. After confirming that intermittent fasting is suitable for your health, the next thing to do is plan how to ease into the habit. In other words, before you fully implement any intermittent fasting regimen, it is a good practice to first test the waters, so to speak, with a less strict form of fasting. Doing this will help your body acclimate to the changes before going into the proper regimen.

Don't Fuss Over What You Can Eat

One common mistake people make when fasting is obsessing over the fasting hours and what to eat when they are finally allowed. Of course, if your fasting window is too small, you are not likely to see any result. Also, don't get too tied up in every little detail of intermittent fasting. For example, you don't have to become too worried because you missed a day. Remember that fasting intermittently should be a lifestyle change if you want to continue to reap the benefits. And for a lifestyle change to be sustainable, you must be able to adapt and use it in a way that even if you face challenges, you will work your way around them somehow. Missing a day or cutting your fast short for reasons beyond your control shouldn't get you worked up and worrying about whether you can do the entire plan. Don't give up.

Again, some people focus too much on what they can eat or not eat. For example, "Can I add just a little butter or cream?" "Would it hurt to eat this type of food during the fasting window?" If your focus is on what you can have or eat while you are fasting, you are giving your attention to the wrong things and putting your mind in an unhelpful state. Give your mind the right focus by concentrating on doing a good, clean, fast, and try to consume only water, tea, or coffee during the window.

Watch Electrolytes

Your body electrolytes are compounds and elements that occur naturally in body fluids, blood, and urine. They can also be ingested through drinks, foods, and supplements. Some of them include magnesium, calcium, potassium, chloride, phosphate, and sodium. Their functions include fluid balance, regulation of the heart and neurological function, acid-base balance, oxygen delivery, and many other functions.

It is important to keep these electrolytes in a state of balance. But many people who practice fasting tend to neglect this and run into problems. Here is a common notion: "Don't let anything into your stomach until the end of your fast" Even those just starting to fast know it doesn't work that way, and they tend to forget or fully stay away from liquids during their fasting window.

When you lose too much water from your body through sweating, vomiting, and diarrhea, or you don't have enough water in your body because you don't drink enough liquids, you increase the risk of electrolyte disorders. It is not okay to drink tea or black coffee throughout the morning period of your fast window. The longer you fast without water, the higher your chances of flushing out electrolytes and running into trouble. You can end up raising your blood pressure, develop muscle twitching and spasms, fatigue, fast heart rate or irregular heartbeat, and many other health problems.

On the other hand, drinking too much water can also tip the water-electrolyte balance. So you want to drink adequate amounts of water and not excess water, whether you are fasting or not.

Give the Calorie Restriction a Rest

Remember that intermittent fasting is different from dieting. Your focus should be on eating healthily during your eating window or eating days instead of focusing on calorie restriction. Even if you are fasting for weight loss, don't obsess over calories. Following a fasting regimen is enough to take care of your calories. It is absolutely unnecessary to engage in a practice that can hurt your metabolism. Combining intermittent fasting with eating too little food in your eating window because you are worried about your calorie intake can cause problems for your metabolism.

One of the major reasons that people push themselves into restricting calories while fasting is their concern for rapid weight loss. You need to be wary of any process that brings about drastic physical changes to your body in very short amounts of time. While it is okay to desire quick results, your health and safety are more important. When you obsess or worry that you are not losing weight as quickly as you want, you are not helping matters. Instead, you are increasing your stress level, and that is counterproductive. You are already taking practical steps toward losing weight by intermittent fasting. Why would you want to undo your hard work by unnecessary worrying?

Simply focus on following a sustainable intermittent fasting regimen and let go of the need to restrict your calorie intake. Intermittent fasting will give your body the right number of calories it needs if you do it properly.

The First Meal of the Eating Window Is Key

Breaking your fast is a crucial part of the process because if you don't get it right, it could quickly develop into unhealthy eating patterns. When you break your fast, it is important to have healthy foods around to prevent grabbing unhealthy feel-good snacks. Make sure what you are eating in your window is not a high-sugar or high-carb meal. Instead, I recommend that you consider breaking your fast with something that is highly nutrient-dense such as a green smoothie, protein shake, or healthy salad.

As much as possible, avoid breaking your fast with foods from a fast-food restaurant, and eating junk foods after your fast is a quick way to ruin all the hard work you've put in during your fasting window. If, for any reason, you can't prepare your meal, ensure that you order very specific foods that will complement your effort and not destroy what you've built.

Break Your Fast Gently

It is okay to feel very hungry after going for a long time without food, even if you were drinking water all through the fasting window. This is particularly true for people who are just starting with fasting. But don't let the intensity of your hunger push you to eat. You don't want to force food hurriedly into your stomach after going long without food, or you might hurt yourself and experience stomach distress. Take it slow when you break your fast. Eat light meals in small portions first when you break your fast. Wait for a couple of minutes for your stomach to get used to the presence of food again before continuing with a normal-sized meal. The waiting period will douse any hunger pangs and remove the urge to rush your meal. Drink some water, and then after about five more minutes, you can eat a normal-sized meal.

Nutrition Is Important

Although intermittent fasting is not dieting and does not specify which foods to eat, limit, and completely avoid, it makes sense to eat healthily. This means focusing on eating a balanced diet, such as:

1. Whole grains
2. Fruits and vegetables (canned in water, fresh, or frozen).
3. Lean sources of protein (lentils, beans, eggs, poultry, tofu, and so on).
4. Healthy fats (nuts, seeds, coconuts, avocados, olive oil, olive, and fatty fish).

It simply doesn't make any sense to go for 16 hours (or more) without food and then spend the rest of the day eating junk. Even if you follow the 5:2 diet and limit your calorie intake to only 500 calories per day for two days, it is totally illogical to follow it with five days of eating highly processed foods and low-quality meals. Combining intermittent fasting with unbalanced diets will lead to nutritional deficiencies and defeat the goal of fasting in the first place. Realize that intermittent fasting is not a magic wand that makes all poor eating habits vanish in a poof! For the practice to work, you must be deliberate about the types of food you eat.

Chapter 14. FAQs

Is an Intermittent Fasting Diet the Right Choice for Me?

So, does an intermittent fasting diet work when compared to other diets? The answer here is a resounding yes. For example, using a 16 hour fast will keep your body burning fat for most of every day! And getting all of your calories during a relatively small eating window stops your body from going into starvation mode and desperately hanging onto body fat. Compared to a normal reduced-calorie diet, this is a huge difference. While any reduced-calorie approach will initially lead to fat loss, your body is an efficient machine

Is an intermittent fasting diet restrictive? Any diet, by its very nature, involves making better food choices. Run a mile if someone tries to sell you on the pancake diet! Eating rubbish can never be a good choice. However, most diets will have you try to eat clean all the time. This is very hard to do and is directly linked to finding yourself eating 12 doughnuts in one sitting after a couple of weeks of deprivation! Intermittent fasting also involves healthy food choices, but it does give you more wiggle room. It is difficult to eat too much junk in a small eating window after you have already had your healthy food. However, it does let you eat enough to stop you from falling off the wagon.

Perhaps the real advantage of intermittent fasting is that it can be a lifestyle rather than a short-term approach. Even if you do manage to follow them long enough to get results, most diets tend to be followed by a rebound-that is, a return to poor eating and fat gain. By viewing fasting as a long-term solution, this problem effectively disappears.

Should I Take Vitamins When I Intermittently Fast?

It is more important than ever to take vitamins and supplements when fasting, as you are skipping meals that were helping to supply you with these vital nutrients, and it's important that you replace them. The biggest problem with vitamins and fasting is that taking a vitamin pill in a fasted state may result in stomach pain, nausea, and diarrhea. To avoid these unpleasant, unsettling effects, try and get your vitamins down while in the fed state. If this is impossible, try taking your vitamins at night so you can sleep through the discomfort.

Alternatively, you might choose vitamins in liquid form, as they are easier to digest while fasting. If you don't normally take vitamins, a basic multivitamin that provides 100% of your daily intake is a great start to ensure you aren't missing out on anything while intermittently fasting.

Why Would Anyone Fast Who Doesn't Want to Lose Weight?

It might appear to be odd to somebody who is thinking about irregularly fasting to get thinner, for any individual who has their weight leveled out to change their dietary patterns or examples. All things considered, would they say they aren't now experiencing the fantasy? We should not disregard the wide range of various advantages of irregular fasting:

- Fasting for health benefits: Some people swear by fasting because they feel it improves their sleep, mental clarity, and helps them control and maintain chronic diseases such as diabetes, cardiovascular disease, multiple sclerosis, fibromyalgia, and chronic fatigue syndrome, cancer, and the side effects from chemotherapy.
- Fasting for athletes: Fasting offers a consistent method of fueling and resting the body that works under many of the same principles as training and rest days. It offers them a much more convenient way to ensure that they consume the food they need to train than the other option of eating small meals every 2 or 3 hours, and it allows them to maintain a nutrition routine that provides a lengthier feeding time which can be enjoyed with friends and family.
- Fasting for busy people with poor eating habits: People who travel a lot for business often feel less than well most of the time due to poor eating habits developed due to airport restaurants and late-night vending machines.
- Make sure you are well-hydrated and avoid salty or sugary foods before you fast.
- Don't stuff yourself the night before your fast. This "last supper" mentality is a rookie mistake that will give you indigestion, a poor night's sleep, and an even ruder awakening to your stomach and brain when you follow up the preceding evening's bacchanalia with a fasting period.

Why Do I Get Headaches When I Fast, and How Can I Stop Them?

Complaints of headaches, especially when beginning an intermittent fasting program, are quite common. If you are waking with a headache, you may not have hydrated yourself enough the night before.

Isn't Intermittent Fasting Just a Fancy Way of Saying I'm Starving Myself?

- The body uses fatty acids as an energy source for muscles. Fatty acids also include a chemical called glycerol that can be used, like glucose, as an energy source, but it too will eventually run out.

- Fat stores are depleted, and the body turns to stored protein for energy, breaking down muscle tissue. The muscle tissue breaks down very quickly. When all sources of protein are gone, cells can no longer function.
- The body does not have the energy to fight off bacteria and viruses. It takes 8 to 12 weeks to starve to death, although there have been cases of people surviving 25 weeks or more.

Is Intermittent Fasting Safe for Women?

Women are more hormonally sensitive than men. Because of this, they may respond more intensely to the challenges of intermittent fasting and need to consult with a medical professional before starting an intermittent fasting program, especially if they have menstrual and fertility issues. Once intermittent fasting has been undertaken, women should also pay special attention to their menstrual cycle and seek medical guidance if they begin missing periods.

There is a modified technique of intermittent fasting that will help women who experience hormonal sensitivity. In addition, this more progressive approach will help the female body adapt to fasting.

- Fast for 12-16 hours
- On fasting days, stick to light workouts such as yoga or light cardio.
- Drink loads of water
- Save strength training for feeding periods or feeding days

Why Can't I Have a Protein Shake When I'm Fasting?

You can't eat food when you are intermittently fasting – hence you can't drink a protein shake. People get confused about protein shakes – check out diet, fitness, nutrition, and health websites if you don't believe me.

If you are on a 5:2 type of intermittent fasting program and you are consuming 500 to 600 calories on your "low" days, feel free to indulge in one or 2 of these shakes if they don't bring you over your total calorie count. Don't even think about it if you are on Whole Day Fasting or in the fasting portion of your time-restricted intermittent fasting cycle!

Chapter 15. Steps to Follow in Intermittent Fasting

"Beginning is the hardest but is worth it at the end," unknown.

With the spirit of the above quote in mind, let's begin a step-by-step guide on exactly how to fast intermittently.

Step 1: Get Clear on Your Goals

Having clear goals can generally take you far in life, but don't underestimate the importance of defining your objectives before starting an IF regimen.

It was losing the excess weight I had put on during and after pregnancy (this consequently solved a bunch of other health issues for me), improving metabolic health, and achieving mental sharpness and focus. Broadly speaking, I wanted to experience overall better health for my own sake and, most importantly, my baby's. However, my research indicated that I needed to define exactly what I wanted out of IF to reap its full benefits.

And let me explain why this is the case.

Defining your goals when it comes to IF is critical for several reasons. First and foremost, it allows you to pick the most suitable IF method that will effectively take you closer to what you want. For instance, the Alternate-Day IF method is more fitting for those aiming to lose weight, while the 16:8 method is more of a healthy lifestyle change.

While weight loss is one of the most popular reasons people embark on an IF journey, find out what you want out of the diet and then move to the step below.

Step 2: Choose Your Method

Now that you know exactly what you're seeking from IF, the next step involves picking a suitable IF method that will help you achieve your goals.

In addition to your specific goals regarding IF, other factors also go into choosing an IF method that would yield the most benefits for you. These include the length of time you want to fast, your daily routine, what field you work in, what a typical workday looks like for you, the specific climatic conditions prevailing in your part of the world, and how often you dine out with friends and family—to name a few.

Once you have chosen an IF method, though, remember that you're not stuck with it forever. It is completely possible to transition from one type of IF to another if you find that your current regimen isn't working for you or if you think you've mastered the moderate forms of IF (think of the 16:8 method) and want to go pro and explore some relatively challenging routes such as the alternate-day fasting.

Besides, a person should give at least one month's serious go to any particular IF method before quitting or switching it up for good.

Step 3: Identify Your Calorie Needs

While IF is naturally designed to create a calorie deficit when you're fasting, this can be quickly turned into a surplus if you're not mindful of the calories you consume during your eating windows.

Some people practicing IF are usually the least concerned about counting and measuring their calories. Although keeping track of one's calorie consumption is important to a certain extent (even while fasting intermittently), these folks think that their calorie consumption is automatically taken care of as a direct result of fasting intermittently. While this may work out well for someone who doesn't suffer from (or is prone to) an eating disorder such as anorexia, orthorexia, and binge eating, it can be detrimental for individuals whose eating disorders may be triggered by IF.

Keeping track of the number of calories you consume during IF is also important because even if certain methods of IF, such as the Alternate-Day fasting, do allow for calorie consumption during fasting days, there is a limit to how much of these calories one can consume. Again, this restriction is meant to facilitate the benefits of IF, such as weight loss.

Besides, there is a popular opinion that as long as you consume just under 50 calories in the morning, you will be considered to be in the fasting state. This can be critical for those practicing the 16:8 method by having an early dinner and delayed breakfast in an attempt to reach a 16-hour milestone with their fasting. Such people can drink plain water or have a cup of black coffee (no added sugar!) without the risk of breaking their fast in the mornings.

But, guess what, this also implies that you have to be mindful of the calories you consume to ensure that your IF regimen is not wasted.

All of this leads to one conclusion. Whether you're fasting or feasting, you must keep an eye on your calorie consumption to achieve your goals with IF. At least in the beginning.

There are several applications available today that can be used to monitor calorie intake. Some of the best ones include "MyFitnessPal" and "Lose It," which include a calorie counter and boast a food diary and an exercise log.

As you get the hang of doing IF in any way or form that you think best suits you and your situation, the focus on calorie intake will usually wind up fading into the background as IF and your new eating habits get ingrained into your schedule. You will find that you do not need to track the calories as much because you know the approximate amounts which y daily. This is when the much-vaunted benefit of not needing to count calories comes back straight into play, with a vengeance! Because you have more practice and have already established a fair routine and habit of doing you IF lifestyle, your daily caloric intake is more or less at your fingertips. Consequently, you end up not paying too much attention to that, as you can carry on with your daily stuff without worrying about the calorie count.

Step 4: Conduct Meal Planning Without Overdoing It

And no. I'm not about to contradict myself here.

IF is quite liberating in the sense that it allows one to let go of the tedious job of meal planning all the time.

And I'm not going back on my words here.

This step is, in fact, pretty optional. You have the choice of doing it or not.

IF is not a practice meant to put restrictions on someone when it comes to what they eat.

Nonetheless, we all know that a balanced and nutritious diet is critical for maintaining good health, regardless of whether or not you practice IF.

One thing that must be understood is that restricting food for a certain number of hours does not justify consuming junk food when the eating window finally opens. Making unhealthy food choices when you finally sit down to eat in an IF regimen is detrimental to your overall health and will also put any and all of your efforts with regard to IF go to waste.

And you don't want that.

As a result, it's a good idea to set aside some time to (informally) prepare your meals for the coming week. This will not help you keep track of your calorie intake (and thereby lose and maintain weight consistently) but also ensure that you have everything you need to cook a healthy, nutritious and delicious meal on hand.

Because let's be honest, we are more susceptible to ordering takeaway food, and eating unhealthy snacks when prepping a healthy meal at home becomes difficult due to any reason.

And frankly, if you find yourself eating loads of unhealthy food when you aren't fasting, you might as well not fast at all!

Step 5: Begin Your IF Journey with the Pedal to the Metal

Once you have completed all of the steps above, you are now ready to begin your IF journey and see where it takes you.

Along with all of my very best wishes, here are a few things that I would like you to keep in mind while you're at it:

- Make the calories count in the beginning by keeping the nutritional value of any food you consume in insight.
- Practice moderation, both while fasting and feasting.
- Take IF as an opportunity to improve your eating habits and food choices. Fewer meals mean more time for preparing healthy food to dine on.
- IF isn't a one-size-fits-all approach, so keep experimenting to figure out what works best for you.

Chapter 16. Myths About Intermittent Fasting

There are many myths about intermittent fasting. Let's talk about the most typical, especially concerning fitness.

If you want to gain muscle mass in the world of fitness, you have to make many meals to accelerate the metabolism, incorporate protein in each of them, and do not forget to drink your post-workout shake.

Of course, many fitness gurus will never recommend you perform fasting workouts for the possible loss of muscle mass, so let's shed some light on it.

Fasting Periods Reduce Metabolism

In general, there is an excessive and irrational fear that our metabolism will slow down. However, in this book on the reverse diet and metabolic tomb, we have already seen the real impact of caloric restriction and weight loss on metabolism.

Performing fasting periods does not reduce our basal metabolism. Yes, throughout life, it has been repeated that if you skip breakfast, your metabolism is reduced, your body goes into saving mode, and you will accumulate body fat.

But this statement is false. Skipping breakfast does not reduce metabolism.

On the other hand, in several studies, it has been observed that fasting does not reduce metabolism either. In fact, in this study, it was observed that fasting increased the levels of norepinephrine, a catecholamine with different physiological functions, increasing metabolism.

Another reason for criticizing intermittent fasting is the frequency of meals.

Some people say that intermittent fasting is not a good option to lose body fat because the number of made meals is reduced, which can hurt metabolism.

We know that there is no difference between making 3 or 6 meals when losing body fat. This study also concludes that making more meals a day does not translate into a greater loss of body fat.

On the other hand, some studies conclude that alternating fasting days is more effective for losing weight than traditional caloric restriction. In contrast, it has been observed that in others, it is not superior after one year of follow-up.

The nutritional strategy to follow depends on the person. As always, you have to individualize, and some people will adapt better to fasting so that the results will be better.

But it must be made clear that fasting does not reduce metabolism. In any case, the short-term impact would be positive.

Fasting Causes Loss of Muscle Mass

Fasting reduces your basal metabolism and makes you lose muscle mass, as many keep repeating today.

Although caloric restriction (especially if the caloric deficit is very aggressive) can lead to a loss of muscle mass, this loss of muscle mass will be greatly reduced if we include strength training and enough protein in the diet.

If we add the fast to this equation, the result remains the same. However, if you perform heavy strength workouts, include enough protein in your diet, and control the calories you are consuming, the loss of muscle mass will be minimal.

In different studies, it has been observed that it is possible to lose body fat and maintain muscle mass while following a fasting protocol.

In people who practice Ramadan (with experience in training), there is a loss of body weight, but not muscle tissue.

Fasting Increases the Feeling of Hunger So That You Will Eat More

In many studies, there has been an increase in the feeling of hunger.

That is, in general, fasting does seem to increase the sensation of hunger. Still, it has not been observed that this contributes to an increase in caloric intake throughout the day. The opposite has been observed. Performing 1 day of fasting translates into a 30% reduction in caloric intake for the next 3 days, 30%.

Besides, in my personal experience, there is a period of adaptation. The feeling of hunger is reduced as you practice more intermittent fasting. My recommendation is that while you do it try to be active and do things, some exercise is fine, although if you are starting, it is better to start progressively.

Fasting Improves Athletic Performance

Another of the supposed benefits is that performing fasting workouts improves athletic performance.

The reality is that there is no scientific evidence to affirm that fasting improves athletic performance. The studies available today contradict this claim. Training on an empty stomach is not a strategy Useful for improving performance.

In fact, and it is important to mention it, in these studies, the maximum that is achieved is to maintain the performance, and not always since in several the sports, performance is reduced (although it could be due to other factors).

What Happens When You Don't Eat For 24 Hours? Myth Vs. Reality

Myth 1: Your Metabolism Slows Down

This idea has its origin in studies with mice, but there are two problems:

A mouse has a short life (2-3 years). A fast of a day in a mouse would perhaps equal more than a week in a human.

Mice have very little fat and are more sensitive to caloric deficits. On the contrary, humans are mammals with more% fat.

Interestingly, in us, fasting causes a slight increase in metabolism, partly because of the release of norepinephrine and orexin. It is an evolutionary adaptation: motivation to go hunting.

Of course, a prolonged fast will slow the metabolism. It is logical, knowing that leptin takes several days to reduce enough hypothalamus to react, regulating downward energy expenditure.

As we saw in this book, what slows down the metabolism is precisely a prolonged period of a hypocaloric diet, just what they recommend.

Myth 2: Burn Muscle

When your body has consumed all the amino acids in the blood and stored glycogen, start using protein stores in your muscles, to convert them into glucose (via gluconeogenesis). You should avoid this process, but fortunately, it does not happen in the first 24 hours of fasting. A couple of examples:

This study concludes that intermittent fasting retains more muscle mass than a traditional hypocaloric approach (with similar fat loss).

Another study with intermittent fasting in obese adults finds that it is effective for weight loss, even increasing muscle mass. This study also compared intermittent fasting with a high-fat approach (45% of total calories) against another moderate in fat (25% of total calories). The high fat achieved greater muscle gain and fat loss. Interesting.

One possible limitation of these studies is that they are performed in overweight people, and we know that fat protects the muscle.

What would happen in people with a lot of muscle and low fat?

According to this study on Muslim bodybuilders, fasting during the month of Ramadan does not result in loss of muscle mass. On the contrary, women who trained strength with intermittent fasting (16/8) gained the same amount of muscle as those who did more meals, but I lost some more fat.

Fasting-induced increases in growth hormone, the protective function of autophagy, and the reduction of myostatin, which prevents muscle production, could all play a role.

Supplement companies invest a lot of money in promoting the need to ingest 20g of protein every 3 hours, not to catabolize. His dream would be for everyone to drink protein shakes as snacks. It is not necessary.

But more is not better. A prolonged fast is dangerous for the muscle. Your tolerance level will depend on the accumulated glycogen and physical activity performed, but in general, I do not recommend frequent fasting for more than 24-36 hours. Runaway from detox diets for a week, for example.

Myth 3: Low Sugar

The body is designed to maintain the proper level of blood glucose. When you eat, do you produce insulin to store excess glucose? When you fast, do you produce glucagon to release stored glucose? Eating frequently to control blood glucose externally is not necessary. You can use the time to do something more constructive.

Intermittent fasting helps restore sensitivity to a greater extent than classical calorie restriction in people with insulin resistance.

In another study, people with type II diabetes responded better to two large meals a day than six small ones. We also know that intermittent fasting is effective against metabolic problems.

Myth 4: You Will Not Give Up in Training

The impact of fasting on performance depends on many factors, such as the type of physical activity, the duration of fasting, and the level of adaptation. Still, there are many examples where this loss of performance does not materialize once adopted.

Evaluations of studies on Muslim athletes during Ramadan show inconsistent results. Resistance tests are most affected, but it is necessary to consider that the fluids are also restricted during Ramadan, so it is difficult to know what effect is due to fasting and which is due to daily dehydration. In any case, the variations are small.

The truth is that fasting training (with low glycogen) favors adaptations that would not occur if you always train with full reserves. So here I talk more about the subject.

And finally, a recent study on strength athletes demonstrates that an intermittent fasting strategy maintains muscle performance and gains and is more effective in losing fat. The same concludes this study on women.

Myth 5: You Will Be Hungry, Headaches, And Irritation

All this may happen the first time. Like everything, it is a matter of adaptation.

But there is much evidence against distributing food in many small intakes:

This study concludes that increasing the frequency of meals increases hunger.

Another study suggests that it can promote a higher caloric intake.

My experience: the most important thing to improve adherence (and therefore success) is to be satiated when you eat. If you eat 1,800 calories a day and divide it into 6 intakes, you have 300 calories left over. Result: constant hunger. This study finds that compressing the feeding window reduces appetite.

Regarding irritation, it is subjective, but some studies indicate that intermittent fasting improves mood and symptoms of depression and improves mental alertness.

Personally, it would irritate me much more to have to prepare six meals a day and never be satiated. Intermittent fasting represents great mental and time release.

Myth 6: You Will Gain Weight

Simply absurd. Multiple studies show that intermittent fasting helps you lose fat better overall than classic hypocaloric diets. Recent assessments already recognize it as an effective strategy to lose weight.

The justification of some is that by skipping one meal, you will accumulate hunger, and you will eat twice as much at the next meal, but we know that does not happen.

Chapter 17. Potential Risks of Intermittent Fasting for Women Over 50

Intermittent fasting has continued to receive massive publicity that mainly focuses on the benefits of embracing this lifestyle. But have you stopped to think about the negative effects? Well, like any other diet, intermittent fasting also presents potential negative effects that you need to be aware of before getting into it so that you make informed choices. Here are some of the negative effects of intermittent fasting you need to know before you try the trendy diet plan:

You'll Experience Real Hunger

If you are used to eating every so often throughout the day, then you will have problems with intermittent fasting because you will experience real hunger. You should not give up right away and break your fast when this happens. Instead, take active steps to help you to keep going. For instance, you need to make sure you stay away from food, including the smell of food, as this can distract you and trigger the release of gastric acid in your stomach, making you feel hungry. You will also do well to make sure you are well-hydrated and distract yourself by reading a book, going to a movie, or going on a walk.

It Has Risks

A lot of what is said about intermittent fasting is the benefits. But you will be surprised to learn that there are risks linked to this pattern of eating. That is why you need to begin by having a conversation with your doctor, especially if you are more than 65 years old and at risk of health complications. Intermittent fasting also puts you at risk if your job involves lifting heavy equipment because you could experience low blood sugar and light-headedness that could endanger the lives of others. Other categories of people at risk and who must stop fasting immediately, include those underweight, pregnant, have diabetes, take medications, have a history of amenorrhea, are breastfeeding, have an eating disorder, struggle with perfectionism, or struggle with perfectionism have mood instability.

It Could Result in Disordered Eating

Although there is little documentation of intermittent fasting in humans, this eating pattern is likely to develop eating disorders. This is because of the impending temptation to overdo the fast and feast, which eventually negates the benefits you could have already achieved. This is dangerous in the long run because you can get stuck in the cycle.

It Is Not a Realistic Long-Term Solution

Just as it is with many other diets, sticking to intermittent fasting can be difficult in the long run. Research comparing intermittent fasting to other every day caloric restriction diets found that those who practiced intermittent fasting had a higher rate of dropouts than those who practiced calorie cutting. However, the most interesting finding of this study is that the majority of those assigned to the fasting community actually decreased their calorie consumption.

Impaired Performance in Athletes

If you're an athlete, you'll want to eat to get the most out of your workout at the right times. As a result, calorie restriction for long periods can impair your results. This will leave you feeling too sluggish even to push the pedal and claim the medal. If you don't time your workout to coincide with your feasting window, you will also miss out on muscle growth and glycogen replenishment. As a result, you will end up breaking down your metabolism-boosting muscle instead of building it.

You May Have Cravings

Most of the intermittent fasting protocols will require you to go for long periods without food. The only thing you are free to take is water and unsweetened coffee and tea. Ironically, cravings tend to kick in when you are restricted from eating certain foods. You will be surprised at how likely you crave refined carbs and sweets just because your body requires the glucose hit. You will do well to distract yourself from thinking about food during your fasting window. You can also consider indulging a little during the feeding window so that you satisfy those cravings.

Irritability

It's common to feel a little cranky because of a drop in your blood sugar levels. Unfortunately, this can get worse when coupled with other side effects like low energy and cravings. The best way to deal with this is by avoiding people or situations that are likely to make you feel more annoyed and instead focusing on the things that will make you happy.

Feeling Cold

When you fast, your blood flow to your fat stores increases, resulting in cold toes and fingers. This is known as adipose tissue blood flow, and it's essential for moving fat to your muscles, where it's burned for energy. A decline in your blood sugar levels may also be responsible for the increased sensitivity to cold. You can combat this feeling of coldness with hot showers, sipping hot tea, or dressing up in layered clothing. Where possible, stay indoors for longer.

Constipation, Heartburn, and Bloating

When you eat, your stomach releases acid that is vital in aiding digestion. This means that when you are not eating, you could experience heartburn because there is no food for the acid to act on. Other related complications include burping and mild discomfort. You could also experience pain. These signs and symptoms normally go away with time. When it's time to eat, all you have to do now is drink plenty of water and avoid spicy and greasy foods, which are known to aggravate heartburn. See a doctor if it doesn't go down.

Overeating

Most people tend to overeat, especially in the initial days of the intermittent fasting journey. This may be due to the misconception that calories aren't counted while fasting intermittently. Overeating is a product of food excitement. It is important to prepare your meals ahead of time to consume sufficient portions. Even though you may feel famished at the end of the fasting window, try to eat normally.

Overreliance on Coffee and Tea

Most of the intermittent fasting methods you can practice require you to take plenty of water and fluids to stay hydrated and fend off the feeling of hunger. The two most preferred beverages you can take alongside water are tea and coffee. Thus, it is not surprising if you get to a point where you are overly dependent on coffee and tea. Taking too much caffeine can destabilize the quality of your sleep resulting in stress and anxiety that may well promote rebound weight gain.

Feeling Too Full After Eating

When your body gets used to staying without food over lengthy periods, it affects how you process satiety. You will begin to realize that eating any snack or a light meal leaves you feeling too full. This may eventually affect your nutrient intake because then you might end up under-eating.

Intermittent fasting presents some not so awesome side effects that you are likely to experience, especially at the beginning. The secret to coping with these side effects is trying to adjust your fasting schedule. In the long run, you must strike a balance between the benefits and side effects before deciding which way to go.

Chapter 18. The OMAD ("One Meal a Day") Method

OMAD stands for "one meal a day" It is a form of intermittent fasting. This menu helps you prepare OMAD safely and effectively, with enough calories and protein to help you reach your weight loss and low-carb goals.

The OMAD diet is the longest form of a limited-time window diet, equivalent to a 23:1 fast (23 hours of fasting and the ability to eat in a 1-hour time window). The OMAD diet does not impose a specific caloric restriction or macronutrient composition in its purest form. As such, we recommend continuing the healthy low-carb diet during that meal.

Is OMAD Good for Weight Loss?

When the body is in a fasting state, it uses fat reserves as fuel for energy. This leads to the breakdown and utilization of fat. This helps in maintaining lifestyle-related disorders. It also reduces inflammation levels and increases growth hormone (HGH) levels that help burn fat.

Consumption of fibrous fruits and vegetables leads to less absorption of sugar and fat in the body. Fiber also improves digestion and relieves constipation. All of these things collectively lead to weight reduction.

Advantages of The OMAD Diet:

- OMAD diet leads to weight loss: Intermittent fasting and only one meal per day reduce caloric intake, thus promoting weight loss.
- Useful in type II diabetes: Intake of fiber-rich foods with low glycemic index controls blood sugar spikes. Weight reduction also helps reduce hyperinsulinemia.
- Heart-friendly: Reduces visceral fat and improves heart function.
- Feeling light: Intermittent fasting reduces fat deposits in the body, making you more active and less fatigued.
- Induces self-control: The OMAD diet inculcates the habit of selecting nutritious foods. Consciously, with practice, you will overcome your cravings and overeating.

Many of those who eat an OMAD model tend to do so just for the ease of preparing food and eating once a day. This can be especially helpful for those who frequently travel, those on shifts at work, and those with busy schedules.

Think about how much time you spend shopping, planning, and preparing meals. (And let's not even talk about dirty dishes). How much time could you save if there are three meals a day by cutting out two-thirds?

Some people see the OMAD diet as an "easy" way to reduce calorie intake. However, when eating is only allowed for a 30-60 minutes time period, it becomes physically difficult to exceed your daily calorie requirements.

OMAD Diet Side Effects:

- Overeating or bingeing: When you start with OMAD, fasting for 23 hours may cause you to choose unhealthy food options. You get uncontrollable cravings for junk food and desserts. This gets better with time as your body begins to accept the routine.
- Hypoglycemia: There is always a risk of a lack of energy. In severe cases, the person may go dark. Other symptoms include constant hunger, fatigue, shaking, inability to concentrate, and irritability. This also improves with time.
- Consistency: Calorie restriction will initially cause weight loss. But it is difficult to stick to this routine permanently. So, this may lead to weight recycling.
- Physical and Psychological Symptoms: Intermittent fasting increases stress on the body leading to anxiety-related disorders like nausea and mouth ulcers. Acidity can become a problem if your other lifestyle traits are not correct. Ex. Improper sleep and OMAD in combination can lead to acidity and reflux together.
- Sleep Disorder: Intermittent fasting and calorie restriction could affect the central nervous system. This may affect the clarity, focus, and rhythm of sleep.
- Difficult to follow: It takes willpower and fortitude to stick to this diet pattern.

OMAD is definitely not a good option for those who lack motivation and cannot resist temptation.

Foods to Include in The OMAD Diet and To Avoid

You can include:

- **Vegetables:** Green leafy vegetables, carrot, broccoli, cabbage, cauliflower, red beet, lettuce, bell peppers, sweet potatoes, and squash.

- **Fruits:** Apple, banana, orange, grapefruit, grapes, cucumber, tomato, peach, plum, lemon, lime, pineapple, and berries.
- **Animal protein:** White meat such as chicken, lean meat, fish, and eggs.
- **Vegetable proteins:** Legumes, dal, mushrooms, soybeans, tofu, nuts, and seeds.
- **Milk and its products:** Whole milk, curds, cheese, buttermilk, and paneer.
- Whole grains: Brown rice, black rice, cracked wheat, millet, quinoa, and barley.
- **Fats and oils:** Omega-3-rich olive oil, MUFA-rich rice bran oil, sunflower butter, peanut butter, coconut oil, and almond butter.
- **Nuts and Seeds:** MUFA- and PUFA-rich nuts such as almonds, walnuts, pistachios, sunflower seeds, pumpkin seeds, and melon seeds.
- **Herbs and Spices:** Mint, fennel, thyme, oregano, garlic, ginger, onion, coriander, cumin, turmeric, pepper, cardamom, and cloves.
- **Beverages:** Zero-calorie beverages such as water, homemade salted lemonade, green tea, black tea, or sugar-free black coffee.

You cannot include:

- **Fruits consume:** Grapes, Jackfruit, Mango, Chikoo, Sitaphal, and Pineapple in very small amounts.
- **Canned foods:** Canned meats, pineapples, cherries, jams, jellies, or olives as it contains many preservatives, sugar, and salt.
- **Milk and its products:** Low-fat milk and products, flavored yogurt, and cream cheese.
- Grains: with a high glycemic index, such as rice and refined flour, they could lead to weight gain.
- **Nuts and seeds:** Limit consumption of cashews as it could also lead to weight gain.
- **Fats and oils:** Trans fats containing margarine, lard, vegetable oil, butter, and mayonnaise to prevent heart disease.
- **Beverages:** Packaged fruit and vegetable juices, carbonated drinks and energy drinks as it contains simple sugars that lead to weight gain.

Who Shouldn't Follow the OMAD Diet?

- Diabetics on insulin.
- People with severe kidney or liver disease.
- Pregnant and lactating women.
- People who suffer from hyperacidity should avoid OMAD.

Simple Tips for Following the OMAD Diet for Weight Loss

- Keep yourself sufficiently hydrated.
- Start by following the pattern for 1-2 days a week.
- Then gradually increase the number of days until you feel comfortable.
- You can choose the mealtime according to your convenience.
- It is important to eat at the same time every day.
- You can consume 3-4 cups of zero-calorie green tea or spiced teas during the fasting phase.
- Consume an egg or 1 serving of nuts before working out.
- Drink coconut water after your workout to replace electrolytes.
- Get at least 7 to 8 hours of sleep.
- Avoid junk foods and fruit juices.

To Finish About OMAD

The OMAD diet is effective in weight loss and prevents weight regain. But every individual will react differently to the OMAD diet. It will only work wonders if you change a healthy lifestyle. Always consult a qualified professional before trying anything new. The best path to a sustainable life is through a healthy and balanced diet, regular exercise, and a healthy lifestyle.

The Weekly Plan of The OMAD Diet

This menu helps you do OMAD safely and effectively, with enough calories and protein to help you achieve your weight loss and low-carb goals. This plan is recommended to be used for a defined period, as it involves one meal per day (lunch or dinner). It is simple and drama-free. Plus, you'll enjoy delicious and nutritious meals. But, of course, be sure to drink plenty of water (you can also have black coffee and tea). And eat enough salt to minimize side effects like headaches.

Chapter 19. Possible Side Effects of the Diet

Even though we can't overlook the way that irregular fasting has a lot of medical advantages. The earlier mentioned are only a couple of them. There are significantly more favorable circumstances that are extraordinary for the human body and increment the life expectancy of people too. There are likewise some negative effects of intermittent fasting. Any individual who is going to begin irregular fasting at any point shortly has to know both the positive and negative effects of fasting and afterwards choose whether it's advantageous for your body or not.

Anxiety Attacks

Another potential side effect of detoxing through intermittent fasting is the potential for an anxiety attack. This can happen when you are withholding food for an extended time, especially if you are new to intermittent fasting.

An anxiety attack may come upon you because you feel that you are not getting enough nutrition or missing your usual feeding times.

Digestive Distress

Since intermittent fasting has a detoxing component to it, you may experience digestive distress during your first few experiences. This is due to your body flushing out much of the residual matter in your body in addition to simply excreting whatever is still leftover in the digestive tract.

While this is normal to a certain extent, care should be taken if you happen to experience severe diarrhea. This may be especially true if you jump into a fasting period after overeating the preceding day. As long as it isn't anything that you feel abnormal, you can attribute it to the detoxing process. However, if symptoms do not subside, then you may need to seek medical attention at once.

You Might Struggle to Maintain Blood Sugar Levels

Although the intermittent fasting diet tends to improve blood sugar levels in most people, this is not always true for everyone. Some people who are eating following the intermittent fasting diet may find that their ability to maintain a healthy blood sugar level is compromised.

The reason why this happens varies. For some people, not eating frequently enough may encourage this to happen. For others, transitioning too quickly or taking on too intense of a fasting cycle too soon can shock the body that causes a strange fluctuation in blood sugar levels.

You Might Experience Hormonal Imbalances

A certain degree of fasting, especially when you build up to it, can support you in having healthier hormone levels. However, intermittent fasting may lead to an unhealthy imbalance of hormones for some people. This can result in a whole slew of different hormone-based symptoms, such as headaches, fatigue, and even menstrual problems in women.

Again, the reason for the hormonal imbalance varies. For some people, particularly those already at risk of experiencing hormonal imbalances, intermittent fasting can trigger these imbalances. For others, it could go back to what they are consuming during the eating windows. Eating meals that are not rich in nutrients and vitamins can result in you not having enough nutrition to support your hormonal levels.

If you begin experiencing hormonal imbalances when you eat the intermittent fasting diet, you must stop and consult your doctor right away. Discovering where the shortcomings are and how you can correct them is vital. Having imbalanced hormones for too long can lead to diseases and illnesses that require constant life-long attention.

Headaches

A decrease in your blood sugar level and the release of stress hormones by your brain as a result of going without food are possible causes of headaches during the fasting window. Problems may also be a clear message from your body telling you that you are very low on water and getting dehydrated. This may happen if you are completely engrossed in your daily activities and you forget to drink the required amount of water your body needs during fasting.

To handle headaches, ensure you stay well hydrated throughout your fasting window. Keep in mind that exceeding the required amount of water per day may also result in adverse effects. Reducing your stress level can also keep headaches away.

Cravings

During your fasting periods, you might find that you have higher levels of desire than usual. This often happens because you are telling yourself that you cannot have any food, so suddenly, you start craving many different foods. This is because all you are thinking about is food. As you think about food, you will begin to think about the different types of food you like and want. Then, the cravings start.

Early on, you may also find yourself craving more sweets or carbs because your body is searching for an energy hit through glucose. While you do not want to have excessive sugar levels during your eating window, you can always have some, as this is bad for blood sugar. The ability to satisfy your cravings is one of the benefits of eating a diet that is not as restrictive as some other foods are.

Low Energy

A feeling of lethargy is not uncommon during fasting, especially at the start. This is your body's natural reaction to switching its energy source from glucose in your meals to fat stored in your body. So, expect to feel a little less energized in your first few weeks of starting with intermittent fasting. To troubleshoot the feeling of lethargy, try as much as possible to stay away from overly strenuous activities. Spending more time sleeping or relaxing is another way to ensure that your energy reserves are not depleted too quickly. The first few weeks are not the time to test your limits or push yourself.

Foul Mood

You may find yourself being on edge during fasting, even if you are someone who is naturally predisposed to being good-natured. The reason for the feeling of edginess is straightforward. You are hungry, yet you won't eat, and you are struggling to keep your cravings in check; plus, you may already be feeling tired and sluggish. Add all of these to the internal hormone changes due to the sharp decline in your blood sugar levels, and it's no wonder why you may be in such a foul mood. Tempers can easily flare up, and you may be quick to become irritated. This is normal when beginning a fasting lifestyle.

Excess Urination

Fasting tends to make you visit the bathroom more frequently than usual. This is an expected side effect since you are drinking more water and other liquids than before. Avoiding water to reduce the number of times you use the bathroom is not a good idea at all, no matter how you look at it. Cutting down water intake while fasting will make your body dehydrate very quickly. If that happens, losing weight will be the least of your problems. Whatever you do, do not avoid drinking water when you are fasting. Doing that is paving the way for a humongous health disaster waiting to happen. You don't want to do that.

Heartburn, Bloating, and Constipation

Your stomach is responsible for producing stomach acid, which is used to break down food and trigger the digestion process. When you eat frequent meals, unusually large meals, regularly, your body is used to producing high amounts of stomach acid to break down your food. As you transition to a fasting diet, your stomach has to get used to not producing as much stomach acid.

You might also notice an increase in constipation and bloating. People who eat regularly consume high amounts of fiber and proteins that support a healthy digestion process. When you switch to the intermittent fasting cycle, you can still eat a high volume of fiber and protein. However, early on, you might find that you forget to. As you discover the right eating habits that work for you, it may take some time for you to get used to finding ways to work in enough fiber and protein to keep your digestion flowing.

Heartburn may not be a widespread adverse effect, but it sometimes occurs in some individuals. Your stomach produces highly concentrated acids to help break down the foods you consume. But when you are fasting, there is no food in your stomach to be broken down, even though acids have already been produced for that purpose. This may lead to heartburn.

Bloating and constipation usually go hand in hand and can be very discomforting to individuals who suffer from it due to fasting.

Heeding the advice to drink adequate amounts of water usually keeps bloating and constipation in check. Heartburn typically resolves itself quickly, but you can take an antacid tablet or two if it persists. You may also consider eating fewer spicy foods when you break your fast.

You Might Experience Low Energy and Irritability

Until now, your body has been used to having a constant stream of energy pouring in all day long. From the time you wake up until you go to bed, it has been receiving some form of power from the foods you eat. So, when you stop eating regularly, your body grows confused. It has to learn to create its energy rather than rely on the heat being offered to it by the food that you are eating.

Depending on how you are eating, your body may also be growing used to consuming fat as a fuel source rather than carbohydrates. This means that, in addition to losing its primary energy source, it also has to switch how it consumes energy and where it comes from. This can lead to lowered energy for a while. Do things that exert the least amount of energy. If you regularly exercise and work out, reducing the amount you work out or switching to a more relaxed workout like yoga can help you during the transition period.

You Might Start Feeling Cold

As you begin to adjust to your intermittent fasting diet, you might find that your fingers and toes get quite cold. This happens because blood flow towards your fat stores is increasing, so blood flow to your extremities reduces slightly. This supports your body in moving fat to your muscles so that it can be burned as fuel to keep your energy levels up.

You Might Find Yourself Overeating

The chances for overeating during the break of the fast are high, especially for beginners. Understandably, you will feel starving after going without food for longer than you are used to. This hunger causes some people to eat hurriedly and surpass their standard meal size and average caloric intake. For others, overeating may be a result of uncontrollable appetite. Hunger may push some people to prepare too much food to break their fast, and if they don't have a grip on their desire, they will continue to eat even when they are satiated. Overeating or binging when you break your fast will make it difficult to reach your optimal health and fitness goal.

Hunger Pangs

People who start intermittent fasting may initially feel quite hungry. This is especially common if you are the type of person who tends to eat regular meals daily.

If you start feeling hungry, you can choose to wait it out if you have an eating window right around the corner. However, if there is a more extended waiting period or you are feeling excessively hungry, you should eat. Feeling hungry to the point that it becomes uncomfortable or distracting is not helpful and will not support you in successfully taking on the intermittent fasting diet. This is a pronounced side effect of going without food for longer than you are accustomed to.

Chapter 20.Foods to Eat and Avoid in Intermittent Fasting

Because you'll likely want to keep your reproductive and menstrual systems working to their best capacities while you engage in intermittent fasting, you'll have to make sure your dietary choices reflect the health you want to see. Of course, you won't really want to "diet" all that much, as mentioned above. Still, you can make certain healthful changes that allow your body to function at its highest capacity. At the same time, it adjusts to intermittent fasting, sheds that excess weight, and reaches a new and purer energy level than you've ever experienced before.

Here, you will be introduced to concepts and details that will help you eat and drink the things that are best suited to your overall growth and success with intermittent fasting. You'll be shown the pros and cons of the intermittent fasting lifestyle, and you'll be taught tips on how to manage hunger and generally achieve your IF goals.

You should know the best and worst that intermittent fasting has to offer, and you should feel confident that the foods you'll seek during your break from fast will be as health-conscious and supportive as possible, based on the information you've gained. Finally, you should also feel prepared to deal with those "worsts" that IF has to offer. If you're not ready to try intermittent fasting, I'll be incredibly surprised.

Pros and Cons of IF as a Dietary/Lifestyle Choice

On the most basic level (without being too redundant), the pros of switching to intermittent fasting (whether as a lifestyle choice or as more of a simple two-month fasting experiment) include:

- Increased health overall through weight loss, lowered insulin and blood sugar levels, heart health, better muscle mass preservation, increased neuroplasticity, the potential for cancer healing, lower blood pressure and cholesterol, healthier hormone production, longer life, re-started/re-inspired nutrient absorption, reduced inflammation, increased energy, improved mental processing and better access to memory
- An increased overall sense of well-being. Both mentally and as a side-effect of having the body type you want through weight loss
- Eased and regulated menstruation, including lessened period cramps and potential for lessened fertility
- The ability to retain your current diet and caloric intake
- The overall simplicity and ease of starting and maintaining your IF approach, and the versatility and flexibility of IF as a practice

On the flip-side, the cons associated with intermittent fasting (as both a lifestyle and momentary dietary choice) include:

- Potential for increased headaches. These are often caused by dehydration and salt withdrawal from eating less than normal. Increase your water intake and mix in a quarter-teaspoon of salt with each water glass, and you'll feel right as rain in no time.
- Potential for constipation. Just increase your fiber intake to help with this issue!
- Potential for dizziness when in a fasting period
- Potential for muscle cramps. Take supplemental magnesium or sit for a while in an Epsom salt bath to cure these "growing" pains.
- Potential for worst-case-scenario side-effects. This potential is only a concern if IF is not practiced the right way for you and your body. Potential side effects include irregular or ceased menses, hair loss, dry skin/acne, slow healing of injuries, mood swings, super-slow metabolism, constant cold feelings, insomnia, etc.
- Potential to binge when you do eat. Be conscious of your body and what it can handle!
- Interference with social eating patterns. It might feel awkward not to eat with everyone else or explain yourself every time you don't.
- Low energy or unproductivity during fast periods this issue can be helped with practice and eating the right types of foods when you eat.
- Some of the lasting effects of IF are still largely unstudied or uncertain, such as its effects on the heart, fertility, breastfeeding women, stress, etc.

What do Foods and Liquids do?

When you go about your first round of intermittent fasting, you'll need to know what to avoid and what to keep close at hand. The following portion will reveal exactly what's safe, what to avoid, and what does what for you.

When it comes to foods, the best things to have around are:

- All Legumes and Beans – good carbs can help lower body weight without planned calorie restriction
- Anything high in protein – is helpful in keeping your energy levels up in your efforts as a whole, even when you're in a period of fasting
- Anything with the herb's cayenne pepper, psyllium, or dried/crushed dandelion – they'll contribute to weight loss without sacrificing calories or effort
- Avocado – a high-, good-calorie fruit that has a lot of healthy fats
- Berries – often high in antioxidants and vitamin C as well as flavonoids for weight loss
- Cruciferous Vegetables – Broccoli, cauliflower, brussels sprouts, and more are incredibly high in fiber, which you'll definitely want to keep constipation at bay with IF
- Eggs – high in protein and great for building muscle during IF periods
- Nuts and Grains – sources of healthy fats and essential fiber
- Potatoes – when prepared in healthy ways, they satiate hunger well and help with weight loss
- Wild-Caught Fish – high in healthy fats while providing protein and vitamin D for your brain

When it comes to liquids, some of it is pretty self-explanatory:

- Water. It's always good for you! It will help keep you hydrated, provide relief with headaches or lightheadedness, or fatigue, and clear your system during the initial detox period. Try adding a squeeze of lemon, some cucumber or strawberry slices, or a couple of sprigs of mint, lavender, or basil to give your water some flavor if you're not enthused with its taste plain.
- If you need something other than water to drink, you can always seek out:
- Probiotic drinks like kefir or kombucha. You can even look for probiotic foods such as sauerkraut, kimchi, miso, pickles, yogurt, tempeh, and more!
- Probiotics work amazingly well at healing your gut, especially in times of intense transition, as with the start of intermittent fasting.
- Black coffee. Try black coffee whenever possible, in moderation.
- Sweeteners and milk aren't productive for your fasting and weight loss goals.
- Heated or chilled vegetable or bone broths
- Teas of any kind
- Apple cider vinegar shots. Instead, try water or other drinks with ACV mixed in.

Drinks to avoid would be:

- Regular soda, diet soda, alcohol, or any high-sugar coconut and almond drinks, i.e., coconut water, coconut milk, almond milk, etc. Go for the low-sugar or unsweetened milk alternative if it's available.
- Anything with artificial sweetener. Artificial sweeteners will shock your insulin levels into imbalance with your blood sugar later on.

Managing Hunger and Other Useful Tips

A few supportive tips to help troubleshoot, keep inspired and stay focused as you may happen to encounter the "cons" of intermittent fasting are as follows.

Generally, keep these pointers in mind: don't over-exercise and over-limit yourself with calorie intake or with food when you do breakfast. Take pictures of your progress to help keep the inspiration flowing, try not to binge when you have breakfast, and make sure to do your proper research or check with your doctor to be sure your plan for intermittent fasting is really the right one for you!

When it comes to managing hunger, the best thing to do is think of hunger as a wave passing over you. Sometimes the build-up to that wave seems unbearable, but it will crest and crash eventually, passing completely over and through you. If you wait it out, keep yourself busy, and take a few sips of a drink instead. You'll find that these hunger pangs are bearable and not quite as overwhelming as they were at the start. By the end of the third day, you should have a significantly increased capacity to handle these feelings of hunger.

If you start feeling dizzy or lightheaded, one of two things is likely happening to you. You may be experiencing low blood volume, or you might be experiencing low blood pressure instead. Just drinking water, in this case, might not help you all that much; in fact, if you just drink water, you'll be diluting the number of electrolytes in your system even more, so try mixing a bit of sea salt in your water instead. Frequently, for those who don't experience dizziness or lightheadedness unless they're intermittently fasting, this addition of sea salt to water does the trick. However, some people were liable to feel dizzy or lightheaded before they ever tried IF. For those people (or for those for whom mixing salt into their water doesn't help), taking magnesium supplements can also work well, and if that still doesn't help, the issue could be something else entirely. Possible adrenal weakness, anemia, or low blood sugar would most likely be the cause in this case.

If your period gets lighter or starts to disappear, make sure you're getting enough fat in your diet when you fast! If you have been limiting calorie intake, stop doing that right now, and be sure not to binge (on the opposite extreme). Just eat what you would if you weren't IF or dieting at all. These slight adjustments should help resolve this issue. If not, seek advice from your doctor.

When you notice you've become moodier, you can do a couple of things to help and troubleshoot the issue. First things first, don't open yourself up to negative moods by keeping the information about your eating pattern shift to yourself and people you really trust. Some people will bombard you with questions, hate, or confusion when you tell them about your work with IF, and you should remember that you don't have to tell anyone who you think won't support you.

Second, you can make sure you're not still in the detox period of intermittent fasting! You'll be working through the detox period during the first few weeks, bringing up lots of literal stink and emotional issues to boot. Bear through the trial period and see if that moodiness lingers. If you're still frustratingly and unusually moody after week two is complete, you might just have low blood sugar. Work to counteract low blood sugar through the foods you choose to eat when you have breakfast, and the issue should clear itself up in no time.

Finally, two pieces of advice are left, and they're some of the most important ones to internalize. First, choose a plan that starts small and incorporates your life in its planning! If you sleep for almost 12 hours each night anyway, the 16:8 method might be best for you. If you constantly wake early without much sleep, you might be better off doing alternate-day fasting. Go with what works for your schedule, and things will start off so much smoother than they would otherwise.

Second and lastly, start with one month and be open; see what happens! You're bound to get frustrated and moody after and during the first week but commit to withstand the awkwardness and at least get through the first two weeks to the beginning of week three. Stick with it and wait to see what this unintentional cleanse has in store for you.

Chapter 21. Diet in Menopause

Menopause is one of the most complicated phases in a woman's life. The time when our bodies begin to change and important natural transitions occur that are too often negatively affected, it is essential to learn how to change our eating habits and eating patterns appropriately. In fact, it often happens that a woman is not ready for this new condition and experiences it with a feeling of defeat as an inevitable sign of time travel, and this feeling of prostration turns out to be too invasive and involves many aspects of one's stomach.

Therefore, it is important to remain calm as soon as there are messages about the first signs of change in our human body, ward off the onset of menopause for the right purpose, and minimize the negative effects of suffering, especially in the early days. Even during this difficult transition, targeted nutrition can be very beneficial.

What Happens to The Body of a Menopausal Woman?

It must be said that a balanced diet has been carried out in life, and there are no major weight fluctuations. This will no doubt be a factor that supports women who are going through menopause, but it is not a sufficient condition to present with classic symptoms that are felt, which can be classified according to the period experienced. In fact, we can distinguish between the pre-menopausal phase, which lasts around 45 to 50 years, and is physiologically compatible with a drastic reduction in the production of the hormone estrogen (responsible for the menstrual cycle, which actually starts irregularly.) This period is accompanied by a series of complex and highly subjective endocrine changes. Compare effectively: headache, depression, anxiety, and sleep disorders.

When someone enters menopause, estrogen hormone production decreases even more dramatically. The range of the symptoms widens, leading to large amounts of the hormone, for example, a certain class called catecholamine adrenaline. The result of these changes is a dangerous heat wave, increased sweating, and the presence of tachycardia, which can be more or less severe.

However, the changes also affect the female genital organs, with the volume of the breasts, uterus, and ovaries decreasing. In addition, the mucous membranes become less active, and vaginal dryness increases. There may also be changes in bone balance, with decreased calcium intake and increased mobilization at the expense of the skeletal system. Because of this, there is a lack of continuous bone formation, and conversely, erosion begins, which is a predisposition for osteoporosis.

Although menopause causes major changes that greatly change a woman's body and soul, metabolism is one of the worst. In fact, during menopause, the absorption and accumulation of sugars and triglycerides change. It is easy to increase some clinical values such as cholesterol and triglycerides, leading to high blood pressure or arteriosclerosis. In addition, many women often complain of disturbing circulatory disorders and local edema, especially in the stomach. It also makes weight gain easier, even though you haven't changed your eating habits.

The Ideal Diet for Menopause

In cases where disorders related to the arrival of menopause become difficult to manage, drug or natural therapy under medical supervision may be necessary. The contribution given by a correct diet at this time can be considerable. In fact, given the profound variables that come into play, it is necessary to modify our food routine, both in order not to be surprised by all these changes and to adapt in the most natural way possible.

The drop in estrogen always causes the problem of fat accumulation in the abdominal area. In fact, they are also responsible for most women's classic hourglass shape, which consists of depositing fat mainly on the hips, which begins to fail with menopause. As a result, we go from a gynoid condition to an android one, with an adipose increase localized on the belly. In addition, the metabolic rate of disposal is reduced. Even if you do not change your diet and eat the same quantities of food as you always have, you could experience weight gain, which will be more marked in the presence of bad habits or an irregular diet. The digestion is also slower and intestinal function becomes more complicated. This further contributes to swelling and the occurrence of intolerance and digestive disorders that have never been disturbed before. Therefore, the beginning will be more problematic and difficult to manage during this period. The distribution of nutrients must be different: reducing the number of low carbohydrates, which is always preferred not to be purified, helps avoid the peak of insulin and at the same time maintains stable blood sugar.

Furthermore, it will be necessary to increase the quantity of both animal and vegetable proteins slightly; choose good fats, prefer seeds and extra virgin olive oil, and severely limit saturated fatty acids (those of animal origin such as lard, lard etc.). All this to increase the proportion of antioxidants taken, which will help counteract the effect of free radicals, whose concentration begins to increase during this period. Finally, it will be necessary to prefer foods rich in phytoestrogens, which will help control the states of stress to which the body is subjected, which will favor, at least in part, the overall estrogenic balance.

These molecules are divided into three main groups, and the foods that contain them should never be missing on our tables: isoflavones, present mainly in legumes such as soy and red clover; lignans, of which flax seeds and oily seeds in general, are particularly rich; cumestani, found in sunflower seeds, beans, and sprouts. In addition, calcium supplementation will be necessary through cheeses such as parmesan, dairy products such as yogurt, egg yolk, and some vegetables such as rocket, Brussels sprouts, broccoli, spinach, asparagus, legumes, dried fruit such as nuts, almonds, or dried grapes.

Excellent additional habits that will help to regain well-being may be: limiting sweets to sporadic occasions, thus drastically reducing sugars (for example, by giving up sugar in coffee and getting used to drinking it bitterly); learning how to dose alcohol a lot (avoiding spirits, liqueurs, and aperitif drinks) and choose only one glass of good wine when you are in company, this because it tends to increase visceral fat which is precisely what is going to settle at the level abdominal. Clearly, it is difficult to reach a high carbohydrate quota even by eating lots of fruit as in a traditional diet. However, a dietary plan to follow can be useful to have a more precise indication of how to distribute the foods. Obviously, one's diet must be structured in a personal way, based on specific metabolic needs and one's lifestyle.

Chapter 22."Superfoods" to Eat for Women Over 50 Who Practice Intermittent Fasting

As we age, it's not only our closet and preference in songs that change. After age 30, our metabolism starts to decline progressively, which means we need to be a lot more selective concerning the foods we consume. There's less space for free calories from sweet drinks, treats, and better demand for foods with a high nutrient-to-calorie proportion. At the same time, many individuals establish a higher admiration for healthy and balanced eating as they age. They're also on the quest for multitasking foods that can help reduce blood stress and cholesterol and secure diseases like type 2 diabetic issues.

List of Foods and Drinks

Intermittent fasting comes with many benefits and positive effects that can be reaped by consuming calorie-free food items. This method of weight loss does not rely on how much you eat. It focuses mainly on the time of eating. Although, there is nothing specific regarding the good items that you can have while fasting. But certain food items can help in making the best out of intermittent fasting. Such food items can also help you stay full for a long time. Here, you will find the food items and drinks you can have for the best results.

Food

Lentils

Lentils are well known for their high fiber content. If you can have half a cup of lentils every day, you will be able to fulfill approximately 32% of your body's overall fiber requirement in one day. Also, lentils are rich in iron, which is necessary, especially for women over the age of 50. So, if you are willing to meet the required nutritional requirements while following intermittent fasting, lentils are a must-have for the diet.

Grains

Carbohydrates are essential for our well-being. Carbs are not regarded as an enemy concerning weight loss. In intermittent fasting, you will need to fast for the majority of the day. So, it is important to think strategically about achieving the required mark of calories while not feeling extremely full. Including food items made from whole grains such as crackers, bagels, and whole-grain bread in your diet can help. Food items made from whole grains are easily digestible. They can also provide you with the required fuel for the functioning of the body. Whole grain food items are a great choice if you want to exercise or work out while practicing intermittent fasting. You will get all the required energy.

Berries

Smoothies made from berries form an essential part of the intermittent fasting diet plan. You can have strawberry smoothies in your breakfast to get your daily dose of Vitamin C. You can also consume one cup of strawberries to meet the overall need of Vitamin C. Berries are a great option for fulfilling all your cravings during the period of fasting. You can add other fruits as well as berries while making smoothies. Consuming smoothies can provide you with the goodness of various food items at one time. Including berry smoothies in your diet can help in improving your overall intake of nutrients.

Seitan

Having a balanced amount of protein daily in your diet is very important. If you are not willing to consume animal-derived proteins, you can opt for the alternatives. One such alternative protein source is seitan. It is also known as wheat meat. Seitan is the richest source of protein that we can get from plants. You can bake seitan and have them with a sauce of your choice. No matter what happens, protein intake is necessary for overall health.

Nuts

Nuts can help in readily getting rid of all types of body fat. So, it will be good for you to make some room in the kitchen for including mixed types of nuts. Nuts are also helpful in improving longevity. Additionally, nuts' consumption can help reduce cardiovascular diseases, type 2 diabetes, and many others. If you do not feel like having nuts directly, you can mix them with smoothies.

Papaya

The last final hours of the fasting window are always going to be the most crucial phase. The primary reason is that you will start getting hungry, especially if you are a beginner. It might result in overeating during the eating window, which will lead to weight gain. The chances are high that you might feel bloated and sluggish as you overeat. Papaya comes with a unique enzyme called papain. Papain can easily act upon all the proteins and break them down. Including papaya in your diet can help in easing the digestion process when paired with protein-rich food items. Papaya can also help in reducing bloating.

Potatoes

Potatoes can help in making your diet balanced. They are capable of providing you with quick energy because of their fast digestion process. Many of you might think of potatoes as being high in fat. But that is not the case. You can pair them with something and try not to consume them alone. You can cook them with food items that are rich in protein. Potatoes can also be consumed as a quick snack as you finish your exercise schedule. Our gut comes with certain good bacteria that can help in maintaining a healthy digestive system. Potatoes can help to maintain the good health of the gut bacteria also. Additionally, potatoes can help you in staying full for a long time.

Hummus

Hummus is often regarded as the creamiest and tastiest dip that can be found today. Hummus is a great protein source that comes from plants. Including hummus in your diet plan can help in improving the nutrition content of several staples like sandwiches. You can prepare a tasty sandwich by applying some hummus to your sandwich along with some vegetables. In case you do not want to have packaged hummus, you can prepare it on your own. Keep in mind that the secret ingredients for tasty hummus are garlic and tahini.

Fortified Milk

The required calcium intake for most adults is about 1000 mg every day. You can achieve your daily intake of calcium by having three full glasses of milk every day. However, as the feeding window is effectively reduced in intermittent fasting, the chance of having this much milk might result in being scarce. So, you will need to shift the focus to food items that are rich in calcium content. Fortified milk comes with vitamin D, which can help the body enhance its ability to absorb calcium. It can also help in making the bones stronger. Combining milk with breakfast cereal or smoothies is a great option to improve your daily calcium intake. You can also opt for drinking them alone after your primary meals. In case you do like milk, shifting to non-dairy sources of calcium, such as tofu, can help.

Avocado

After seeing avocado in this food listing, most of you might doubt your mind. However, avocado is a healthy consumable, despite its high calorific value. Avocado comes with monosaturated fat, which can help in keeping you full for a long time. Additionally, avocado also imparts great levels of satiety. Adding some avocado slices to your meals will allow you to stay full for longer if you opt for tough fasting practices. You will also be able to control your food cravings while fasting. Thus, you can effectively prevent yourself from consuming unhealthy food items and snacks.

Fish

According to the latest Dietary Guidelines, including at least eight ounces of fish in your diet every week is necessary. It is definitely for something positive. Fish are rich in proteins and healthy fats. They are rich in vitamin D as well. When you start with your fasting regime, including fish in your diet becomes more important. With only one type of fish, you will be able to provide the body with a full dose of essential nutrients. Additionally, fish can also help in enhancing your brain health.

Cruciferous Veggies

Vegetables like cauliflower, Brussels sprouts, and broccoli come with great fiber content. As you start practicing intermittent fasting, including adequate fiber in your everyday diet is very important. Having cruciferous vegetables can help in dealing with constipation as they are rich in fiber. You can also have the surety of daily bowels. Fiber is well known for providing satiety. So, such vegetables can help you in staying full for a longer period. If you are willing to opt for fasting for 12 – 16 hours, staying full before starting will help provide the best results.

Leafy Greens

Overdoing the spinach, kale, collards, or other leafy eco-friendlies at meals might help to keep your mind sharp as you age. According to a study last month at the American Society for Nutrition annual conference, people who consumed one to 2 servings daily had the same cognitive capacity as people 11 years younger than hardly ever ate environment-friendly ones. Cooking eco-friendlies does not need to be made complex. For a convenient side meal, grab a bag of child spinach and sauté the fallen leaves entirely in a drizzle of olive oil with optional cut garlic.

Heads up: When you take the blood thinner Coumadin, you don't have to surrender eco-friendlies totally; talk to your doctor about adjusting your medicine to enable tiny portions every day.

Drinks

As you start fasting, beverages can help you to stay hydrated for a long time. Also, you will be able to handle your hunger pangs in a better way. While practicing intermittent fasting, there are certain drinks that you can include in your diet.

Tea

Tea is well known for improving satiety naturally. It can act as a secret tool that will make your fasting process easier. It can improve the chances of succeeding in your practice. Various types of tea can be included in your diet while fasting. Some of the common types of tea are green, oolong, herbal, and black. Tea is popular for improving the overall effectiveness of intermittent fasting. It helps in improving gut health, supports probiotic balance, and improves cellular health. Nothing can be as effective as green tea when it comes to weight loss.

Coffee

Including drinks that are free from calories is important for intermittent fasting. If you are willing to include a calorie beverage in your diet, you can opt for black coffee. Normal coffee can also serve the purpose during the window of fasting. Ensure that you do not use sweeteners or milk while having the coffee of your choice. You can try to add some spices to improve the taste of your coffee, like cinnamon. One thing that you will need to do is to keep an eye on your experience of consuming coffee while fasting. It is because many people suffer from racing hearts or upset stomachs right after having coffee while fasting. With coffee consumption, you can keep your levels of blood sugar under proper control without any medication. Coffee can also provide you with a great energy boost while fasting, as the chances are high that you might feel lethargic while fasting.

Water

Water is life. No matter what kind of diet or fasting method you practice, you should always have enough water—drinking plenty of water while fasting can help you to stay hydrated for a long time. If you are tired of having normal water, you can replace the same with sparkling water while fasting. You can also change the taste of water by adding a few lemon juice drops. You are always free to experiment with the flavor of the water. You can infuse a full jug of water with cucumber or orange slices. It will help in making your fasting window fun. However, stay away from using any kind of sweetener in your water. If you use artificial sweeteners with water, it can interfere with the results of the fast.

Chapter 23.Supplements for Intermittent Fasting

Not all supplements can provide the health benefits you need. Taking the wrong supplements, especially while you are on intermittent fasting, may bring harm. The right types of health supplements can significantly boost the effects of intermittent fasting.

We will briefly talk about the problems with taking generic supplements, choosing the right health supplements for those who are into intermittent fasting, and a comprehensive list of health supplements you should take.

The Problem with Multivitamins

Multivitamins are widely used. Since multivitamins are taken by millions of people all over the world, many people believe they are important in the battle against disease and malnutrition. This is, in fact, a misconception. In reality, not everyone can benefit from multivitamins and instead choose targeted supplements.

Nutritional Imbalance

Many multivitamins contain too many specific nutrients, such as Vitamin A or C, and not enough other essential nutrients, such as magnesium. So, there is a tendency to overdose on a few nutrients and not take enough of the others.

Some manufacturers still include a long list of multivitamins on their labels, but the truth is, that some of these vitamins are in very small amounts. Many consumers ignore the insubstantial amounts of important nutrients. How can you fit a range of nutrients in only one pill? Also, we need to consider the nutritional needs of each person. A bodybuilder will require a different set of nutrients compared to a lactating mom.

Low Quality of Multivitamins

Each type of nutrient behaves differently inside the body. While folate is an important B vitamin, folic acid — the form found in generic multivitamins, may increase the risk of colon cancer, according to a study published by the University of Chile.

This could be why some research, such as a 2009 study published by the University of East Finland, suggests a connection between multivitamins and an increase in mortality, while another research commissioned by the American Medical Association in 2009 reveals no benefit in taking multivitamins.

Furthermore, many multivitamins are manufactured with additives and fillers, which make it difficult for the body to absorb nutrients. Therefore, a minimal amount of important nutrients may reach your cells.

We are actually getting what we pay for with multivitamins. You may convince yourself and choose the generic multivitamins in the store, or you may add a bit and choose targeted supplements to help improve your health.

Supplements and Fasting

Eating whole and natural foods is still the best source for getting the important nutrients our body needs. But, remember, whole foods may behave differently from their individual components. For example, the nutrients from a piece of broccoli are more accessible compared to consuming an equal amount of nutrients from a powder or a pill.

The antioxidants sourced from natural foods are beneficial, but consuming mega doses of some synthetic antioxidants may come with risks such as the growth of tumors based on a 1993 toxicology research from the University of Hamburg.

Food synergy enables the nutrients in food to work together. Hence, food is more powerful compared to its components. This is why it is crucial, to begin with, a diet rich in nutrients, then add supplements based on your goals and needs.

It is important to take note that just because something is natural doesn't mean it is helpful. There is a tendency for some, especially the health buffs, to abuse even food-based vitamins and herbal supplements.

These supplements are still vulnerable to contaminants and heavy metals from manufacturing. Be sure to check the sourcing and quality testing of your supplements. It is ideal for checking with a licensed professional who can recommend safe brands of supplements.

Chapter 24. Advantages and Disadvantages of Intermittent Fasting

There are pros and cons to every lifestyle. For instance, when you are eating a healthy and nutritious diet, you may lose weight and gain health but be unable to eat all your favorite foods in the amount you would like. On the other hand, you may enjoy yourself when you eat junk food, but you will lose health and gain weight. In the same way, there are naturally both pros and cons to intermittent fasting, and by understanding what they are, you can better manage your lifestyle.

Like all things, you will find that these pros and cons are most evened out when intermittent fasting is done in moderation. If a person only rarely practices fasting, then they will, in turn, only experience a few of the benefits. Moreover, if they practice intermittent fasting overly enthusiastically and for longer periods than healthy, they will experience more drawbacks.

Thankfully, with a balanced intermittent fasting schedule, you can find yourself experiencing many of the benefits and few, if any, of the drawbacks.

While some pros and cons of intermittent fasting are universal, others can be affected by gender and age. We will be exploring what pros and cons you individually may experience as a woman in or over her fifties.

Advantages of Intermittent Fasting

Boost Weight Loss

Most people discover intermittent fasting either because they want to lose weight or gain health benefits. But, sometimes, losing weight can accomplish both simultaneously, as a high body fat percentage can increase high blood pressure, cholesterol, and early mortality. So, whether you are hoping to gain these health benefits by losing weight or wish to lose weight to feel more comfortable in your skin, you will love the way that intermittent fasting can boost your weight loss.

Balance Important Hormones

Thankfully, studies have found that intermittent fasting can help balance a person's cortisol and melioration levels. It does this in a variety of ways. For instance, it can help to reduce cortisol by balancing and regulating blood sugar levels. Balancing cortisol sets off a chain reaction that improves the balance of other hormones, including melatonin. One simple change can benefit many hormones and systems within your body.

Improve Heart Health

As we age, we all must take even more heart health care. After all, heart disease is the number one killer of both men and women. While most often, doctors educate men on the symptoms and warning signs of heart attacks, women are often forgotten, leading to an increased risk of death. This means women must be extra vigilant, take care of their heart health, and educate themselves on the warning signs of heart attacks.

One crucial way to increase heart health is to watch your cholesterol. There is not a single type of cholesterol, but several. The two main types include LDL, which is known as the "bad" cholesterol, and HDL, known as the "good" cholesterol. While LDL cholesterol will increase your risk of heart attack and heart disease, HDL cholesterol will protect your heart health and remove LDL cholesterol from your body.

Increase Mental Energy and Efficiency

We all need mental energy to get through the day. When our mind is sluggish, we are unable to think, or accomplish anything, and sometimes we may be unable even to stay awake. We have all had trouble at times focusing on work, completing a math problem, remembering what we have read, and so on. This is all due to a lack of mental energy and efficiency. You may think that intermittent fasting would further reduce your mental state, as hunger makes focusing difficult, but it is the exact opposite.

Reduce the Potential Risk of Developing Cancer

Of course, nobody can promise that any lifestyle choice will prevent you from developing cancer in the future. However, studies have found that intermittent fasting can potentially reduce your risk. Further studies are ongoing, but current research through animal studies has proven to be promising. For instance, it was found that rats with tumors survive longer when placed on fasting schedules than the control group.

Increase Longevity

Early studies on animals have found that an animal can experience an increased lifespan by including intermittent fasting. These studies found that even if animals had a higher body fat percentage than the control group, by including intermittent fasting, they were able to increase their lifespan and longevity.

This makes sense, as intermittent fasting has many health benefits, and when all of these benefits are compounded together, it naturally results in a longer lifespan.

Lifestyle Ease

We all want to improve our health and weight, but it is important also to have an easier lifestyle. When it is difficult to gain health and weight, many of us fail, as life is already busy and difficult enough without extra worries and tasks. If a person cooks more, eats more frequently, and always worries about a diet, they are unlikely to stick to it, as it is merely unmaintainable.

It supports the Secretion of the Growth Hormone

It's present in kids more than in grown-ups, but it still helps a lot. The growth hormone decreases fat and improves the development of bones and muscles. It does this by turning glycogen into glucose in the bloodstream. This enables fat burn without the reduction of muscles. When you sleep and exercise enough, the growth hormone is also boosted.

It Enables You to Avoid Heart Illnesses

Both blood glucose control and fat loss are done by intermittent fasting and improve heart health. The likelihood of getting coronary artery heart illness can also be reduced.

Intermittent Fasting Is Very Versatile and Can Fit in Any Schedule

It is not as challenging as certain diets that unnecessarily trigger a huge disturbance in your life. There is no particular time to perform intermittent fasting. They can be combined as you think it is appropriate for your timetable. You are not boxed into any regiment that you cannot retain easily. Intermittent fasting adapts to life's unpredictability. This can also be practiced everywhere in the world as there is no special gear you need to do it; it only restricts your feeding and is therefore much easier and more practical than many diets. It's completely all right, even if you have to halt fasting for a while. In a matter of minutes, you can begin fasting again.

Simple to Practice

Intermittent fasting is easy to do and doesn't have any complicated scheduling. It is quite direct. This causes it to be simpler to pursue and more efficient than many diets.

Opens Up Your Mind

It enables you to regulate your mental procedures as intermittent fasting opens up your body. You are used to responding to your body's urges because you consume whenever you feel slightly hungry. You are released from the control of your body as a result of practicing it.

Improves Your Metabolism

It enhances your metabolism by considerably reducing the number of calories you eat in one day. It is almost possible to eat the suggested daily calorific requirements during the feeding time you have. This causes modifications in the body and fat burning. It also helps you burn fat, even if you eat the normal calories as your system requires, making you burn fat for energy instead of carbs.

Disadvantages of Intermittent Fasting

Getting Started Takes an Adjustment

Any lifestyle change takes an adjustment, and it can take months for something to become a habit. So naturally, intermittent fasting is quite an adjustment for people who are used to grazing on food throughout the day. This means that if you push yourself to go into an advanced version of intermittent fasting when you first begin, you can become overwhelmed. But if you start slowly and allow your body to adjust in its own time, you will find it happens much more naturally and becomes easy to stick to.

Potential to Overeat

While intermittent fasting should naturally reduce caloric intake, if a person pushes themselves to fast when they are overly hungry, it might lead to overeating during their eating window. This is because the person feels hungry for so long when fasting that their body believes it must make up for the calories it lost when they can finally eat. The result is that the person either hits a weight loss plateau or even experiences increased weight.

Possible Leptin Imbalance

The hormone leptin is important as it signals to your body that you are full and that you no longer need to eat. But when a person practices intermittent fasting, it may temporarily disrupt this hormone's production. However, this is usually only a short-term problem, and once a person's body adjusts to their fasting and eating windows, their leptin will balance itself out. Typically, a leptin imbalance is only a real problem when a person dives head-first into intermittent fasting and attempts to practice advanced level fasting when they are still only beginners.

You May Become Dehydrated

Many people do not drink enough water. In general, doctors recommend that we drink half of our body's weight in pounds in ounces of water.

Many people do not drink enough water as it is, but this can make dehydration worse when a person is practicing fasting. This is because fasting boosts the metabolism, and when your cells are in a metabolic accelerated state, they require more water for fuel. If you are not giving them enough water during periods of fasting, you can quickly become dehydrated.

Not only that, but when fasting, you are likely to lose a lot of water weight, which can result in dehydration and a deficiency in electrolytes. Make sure that you drink plenty of water and consume enough electrolytes to prevent this. Thankfully, dehydration is easy to avoid if you remain proactive.

Not Everyone Can Practice Intermittent Fasting

Intermittent fasting is a beautiful and healthy lifestyle for the general population. After all, the human body is designed for practice periods of fasting naturally. However, not every person can practice fasting. Some people, due to chronic illness, may be unable to participate. Ultimately, you must ask your doctor if you are healthy enough to practice short-term fasting.

It Can Trigger the Re-Feeding Syndrome

This hazardous and fatal disorder can happen if you suffer from malnutrition. It is when electrolyte and liquid imbalances occur when malnourished individuals have been hospitalized for a long time and eat again after a long time. The chance of acquiring re-feeding syndrome increases when bodily weight is very small and not eating for more than ten days.

Having Low Energy

Although, after a while, starvation passes, life isn't predictable. You can take part in a tiresome activity that makes you hungry and ultimately unproductive until the hunger goes or you eat. You may have been used to eating a bunch of snacks during the day and quit instantly due to fasting, which may cause a few side effects.

These side effects involve headaches, bad temper, lack of power, constipation, and low concentration levels. It may also decrease your motivation. This sort of fasting can have an adverse fitness effect if you have a health condition. It is not suitable for all. For example, hypoglycemic people require glucose all day, so they can't profit from fasting.

Interfere with the Social Side of Eating

Eating from ancient times was a significant social event. Special times, festivities, milestone accomplishments, and other activities require meal sharing with your friends. Intermittent fasting can mess with your personal life when you change your routine, which may not correspond to the regular eating schedule. On occasions when everyone eats and eats, you may stand out as the one who does not want to participate. Many activities, including dinner meetings, family meals, and romantic meals, are missed, among many others.

Chapter 25. Mistakes to Avoid During Intermittent Fasting

Fasting is not generally seen as a diet, yet a specific way of life and recommended eating schedule. This type of eating plan has increased enormous notoriety as of late, particularly for women over 50. As we have seen, you may fast for 16 hours and eat during an 8-hour window. This is the 16-8 plan and is commonly seen as the standard intermittent fasting plan. A few people follow the alternate day plan, with low-calorie intake on one day and the usual amount the following. Whatever the way you handle it, when your goal is to get in shape, intermittent fasting is famous for one peculiar characteristic: it only works when done correctly.

There are a few potential health benefits when following intermittent fasting. We may include the decreased danger of malignant growth, diabetes, and heart disease among the benefits. Fasting can trigger autophagy, which is known to help with dementia. Regardless of whether you utilize one or another kind of intermittent fasting, it is critical to avoid the traps that can undermine your endeavors. Below are a few intermittent fasting mistakes a lot of people frequently make, especially on their first time.

Looking for too Many Improvements too Fast

You are preparing to begin something new, and you are eager to receive all the rewards as fast as could be. It is normal that you are excited about this new lifestyle and want to dive into it fully. Nevertheless, attempting to get such a large number of improvements too early immediately may disrupt your endeavors.

The key is to begin gradually by including a couple of changes one after another. For instance, if you have chosen to do two 500 calorie days every week while having a regular amount of calories, the other five, consider beginning with only one 500-calorie day. After a couple of weeks, you can feel more confident, including the second day into your weekly schedule.

Not Taking Care of Your Hydration

Staying in a fasting state can be challenging regardless of whether you are not eating. Most drinks will break the fast and extraordinarily diminish any benefits. Although they are fat and calorie-free, it is anything but smart to drink "diet" soft drinks. Indeed, even sugars that have zero calories can negatively influence your insulin levels.

The essential fluid you ought to drink during your fast is water. A moderate amount of coffee will not break your fast, but you will need to take your coffee black in any case. Indeed, even a little sugar in your coffee, like lemon in your water, can influence the fasting period.

Confusing Thirst with Hunger

While it is crucial not to drink inappropriate fluids when fasting, it is similarly essential to ensure you drink enough water. Not getting enough water can make you hungry, and it is anything but difficult to sometimes confuse thirst with hunger.

People get a great deal of water from a good part of their food. Worldwide Food Information states that 20% of the water our bodies use originates from food. This implies that in case you are not eating for a few hours, you will have to drink around 20% more water than usual to compensate for any shortfall.

Eating Unhealthy Foods

Since intermittent fasting is not generally a diet plan, there are not many foods that are "forbidden." This can lead many people to fall into the snare of a binge on junk food the moment their fast is up and the eating time opens. Try not to make an unhealthy eating habit, thinking that fasting will compensate for it.

Make a rundown of all the healthy foods you do appreciate. Do ordinary shopping for food and try to stick to your food decisions. While fulfilling your hunger with not exactly healthy snacks sometimes can be all right, for ideal health and weight-loss achievement, it is important to eat as healthy as possible under the circumstances. Eating the right foods is vital to taking advantage of any weight loss plan. Foods rich in calcium, protein, and vitamin B-12 should be high on your grocery list, particularly for women over 50.

Overeating After Each Fast

This is presumably the greatest trap for both beginners and people who have been fasting intermittently for quite a while. Practicing intermittent fasting to get more fit will lose effectiveness if you end up taking in an excessive amount of calories on every chance you have to eat.

One approach to hold back from overeating is to eat larger amounts of healthier foods during your eating window. This would include heaps of healthy plates of mixed greens and crisp vegetables. It is also a smart idea to arrange meals and prepare seasonings before your fast period starts. Thus, you are not tempted just to grab anything. Finally, remember that it can take as long as about fourteen days until you have changed and adapted to the point that you will not feel that hungry after each fasting period.

Trying to Stick to the Wrong Plan

There are many different approaches to putting intermittent fasting into your daily schedule. For instance, if your fasting plan includes not eating from 8 pm until early afternoon every day and having a challenging activity that begins right in the first part of the day, this is most likely not the correct plan.

What works for one person may not necessarily fit in for another one. To get the most rewards from intermittent fasting, you should take your time to analyze different types of plans thoroughly. It is all right if it takes a little longer to find out the plan that best works for you.

Not Drinking Enough Water

Maybe one of the most common and easily avoidable intermittent fasting mistakes is not taking in enough water.

We know that drinking water is fundamental for overall health, yet it is even more significant when fasting.

Why? Because most of the time, we feel hungry, we are actually dehydrated.

Can you imagine how your hunger might be influenced by lack of water when you are trying to go through the main part of the day without eating?

Fortunately, this is very simple to avoid!

Sneaking more water into your day is as simple as making a couple of basic changes.

A few people truly are bored drinking plain water. Trust me, one thing that may be a great idea is to add a couple of Mio Drops (or other water enhancers) to water. It will have a tremendous effect!

In case you do not know them, Mio Drops are zero-calorie, zero-carb, and sugar-free water enhancers.

Misunderstanding Real Hunger Signs

Perhaps the best thing that I have learned from my intermittent fasting test is that I found a good pace about when appetite shows.

It does not come at 9 am when I've been awake for one hour and last ate a late-night nibble at 11 pm the prior night.

No doubt, your stomach may be growling, and you may desire something yummy.

Yet, you are not really hungry.

Also, it may be wonderful to binge with your family or friends and enjoy the social part of feasting.

Yet, again, you are not really hungry.

Intermittent fasting will teach you that if you stand by fasting long enough, more often than not, your "hunger" will generally blur in no more than five or ten minutes.

It most likely already happened without you noticing or giving it a particular thought.

How many times at work were you planning to go to eat, then some, however, some last-minute rush job showed up, and one hour or two passed by while you overlooked your stomach's protest?

What before looked like the most urgent priority, eating, was overshadowed by something new that popped up. And you survived!

In any case, yielding and eating too early is one of the serious mix-ups with intermittent fasting. Think that by simply drinking some water and allowing it ten minutes or so, you will. Usually, your appetite will calm down.

Try not to break your intermittent fasting plan before you even begin.

Try not to easily give in to bogus hunger!

Is Intermittent Fasting Being Used as an Excuse for Overeating?

One of the most dangerous intermittent fasting errors is succumbing to the urge to think, "What the hell, I've been starving myself all day, I deserve to reward myself for supper!" and then gorge yourself with junk food, filling yourself with unhealthy foods.

Please don't be that woman.

You would feel hopeless and most likely put on weight.

We don't want that.

Although actually, intermittent fasting is not a diet because it does not confine what you eat, it is yet critical to settle on healthier food decisions. You want, most of all, to have a healthy relationship with your food and your body.

Even if you only eat once a day, you can overeat and gain weight if you consume more calories than your body requires.

While you do not need to be an absolute stickler and there is space for adaptability, still be shrewd.

Help yourself out, and do not go crazy during your eating window.

Not Eating Enough

If you have yet to attempt intermittent fasting, the risk of not eating enough during eating times may appear to be illogical.

Actually, for some people, not eating for a particularly long time, it's not unusual to become less hungry.

In some cases, fasting can thoroughly kill your appetite.

Unless you are deliberately doing a total fast (not suggested if not under medical control), however, it is anything but a good idea to decide not to eat enough.

If you should not eat sufficiently for too long, you can easily wreck your digestion and unbalance your hormones.

Furthermore, you can deprive your body of essential nutrients, which can aid in the prevention of health problems that are much more serious than the loss of a few extra pounds.

Consult your physician about a complete, healthy calorie intake that is fit for weight loss and may help you reach your desired outcomes.

Failing to Plan Your Meals in Advance

While calorie tallying is not important (however, truly, you will show more signs of improvement results if you do it), carefully planning and thinking about what you will eat when you're eating period arrives is a great intermittent fasting hack.

This will allow you not to have to improvise when you are finally going to sit down at the table.

Rather than going like, "I'm starving and need to eat now no matter what," and then heading to the closest, cheapest, and more unhealthy junk food, you better learn to tell yourself, "well, I'm feeling hungry now, but I can wait, I'm not dying, and something healthy and delicious is waiting for me, later."

Utilizing this opportunity to consider what you will eat when you eat and sticking to healthier options will only have benefits for you over the long term.

You will learn how to eat for effective weight loss while decreasing caloric intake, keeping you satisfied, and boosting your self-confidence.

If you are fasting for 16 hours, you can easily invest 5 minutes of your time planning what meal will break your fast later.

It is really not unreasonably hard and will prepare for a slimmer future!

Chapter 26. How Does the Woman's Body Change?

The body does not stop changing throughout our lives. Age and genetics are primarily responsible for these changes, although not the only ones. External factors such as tobacco, alcohol, poor diet, or excessive sunbathing are determinants of our health's deterioration over the decades.

In women's case, the number of hormones that we have determines the evolution of our body over the decades. Fertility is also key to understanding the changes that occur. Between the decades of the 20s and 60s, the woman undergoes a series of important changes, both hormonally and physically, as a result of menstrual cycles, pregnancies, and other derivatives of reproductive aging.

At 20 Years Old

During this decade, the woman is full of energy and performance and enjoys a baseline health status. The body adapts to our rhythm of life, and we perform better physically.

Genetics is a fundamental factor that determines endogenous aging; however, everything takes its toll. As much as at 20 years, the skin is full of collagen, a weekend of excesses on the beach or smoking daily are points that accumulate against the epidermis and time. If a person with a genetic predisposition to have a thinner dermis or lighter skin also smokes, sunbathes, and excessive gestures may have wrinkles in the 20s.

Creating good eating and exercise habits while avoiding alcohol and smoking, paying attention to eating disorders, and attending gynecological exams annually.

As for the skin, during this decade and the third, the woman loses the brightness of adolescence and therefore must start using moisturizers, which should subsequently be rich in alpha-hydroxy acids.

During the second decade, the woman is in the fullness of her sexual development by ovarian activity. The secretion of hormones such as estrogen and progesterone plays a fundamental role in the menstrual cycle and fertility.

Our ovaries have a million oocytes at birth and will no longer be produced. In each menstrual cycle, they are discarded, so as time progresses, the possibility of becoming a mother decreases until menopause arrives. Between the ages of 15 and 25, the probability of becoming pregnant in each cycle is 40%. During this time, contraceptive treatments should be taken into account to avoid unwanted pregnancy and assist in the transmission of infectious diseases.

At 30

From the age of 30, there is a decrease in metabolism, which means that we naturally burn fewer calories per minute if we do not exercise.

The specialist Concepción de Lucas points out that your physical condition can worsen if you also lead a sedentary lifestyle, with work stress, or poor diet.

Also, this is the decade in which most Spanish women have their first child: the average is 32 years old. The expert points out that this moment is key for women. "In this decade, muscle tone is lost and, with pregnancy, the body can undergo significant changes, with increases and decreases in weight, body volume, and muscle sagging."

It is also common to observe adult acne, which usually appears in the jaw area and that is due to excessive sensitivity of the skin of that area to hormonal changes and that can be treated with oral contraceptive treatments or oral recurrences (not indicated for pregnant women since it can cause alteration is in the fetus) or synthetic, as dermatologist María Teresa Tracheole explains. This type of acne may also be due to disorders such as the polycystic ovary or the use of overly fatty cosmetics.

From the age of 30, expression wrinkles begin to appear in the areas where we are most gesturing, such as between the eyebrows or the eye area, with bags and crow's feet. The specialist recommends using moisturizers and containing active ingredients such as the alpha as mentioned earlier hydroxy acids, which seek to reshape the skin, vitamin C, and niacinamide.

You have to maintain good eating and exercise habits, go to gynecological exams annually, do health checks to monitor cholesterol, weight, visual and auditory acuity, and early detection of diseases and pathologies.

From the age of 35, the woman's fertility decreases. As a result, it is increasingly difficult to get pregnant, so gynecologists advise not to delay motherhood beyond this age because, in addition to having to resort to assisted reproduction techniques, they add the risks of having abortions, hypertension, diabetes, and deformations or alterations in the fetus. From the age of 40, the probability of pregnancy in each cycle is 25%.

At 40

During the fourth decade of our life, a series of changes in our physiognomy begin to occur. The fat predominated in the buttocks and legs for possible breastfeeding begins to redistribute in the abdomen, increasing cardiovascular disease risk.

Also, decrease muscle mass and tone and increases sagging in arms and legs, especially if we do not exercise.

The level of hormones drops, and the woman is moving away from her period of greatest fertility.

The skin loses elasticity, and sunspots begin to develop like antigens, which are more marked on the lighter skins. As a result, expression wrinkles intensify, and facial volumes begin to vary. The expert recommends anti-spot lasers, botulinum toxin for the expression of wrinkles, and hyaluronic acid to treat the anogenital groove's wrinkles and volume loss.

As Lucas warns, good eating habits and exercise will contribute to a better menopausal transition in the future. The specialist indicates that, from the age of 40, the tendency to suffer from hypertension and cholesterol, pathologies observed in men, rises.

Also, the intervertebral discs are compressed, and it is normal for spine pain, loss of muscle tone to increase, and osteoporosis or loss of bone mass. Young women must prevent their appearance by performing a diet rich in calcium and muscle strength exercises. This serves to condition the muscles and make them stronger and stronger. It also strengthens the union of muscle with a bone through tendons.

From 45 to 50 years old, women can begin to notice hot flashes, irritability, difficulty sleeping, vaginal dryness, decreased libido, and alterations in menstruation; "We are in premenopause," explains Esparza, who advises seeing it as "a natural stage in women," which must be normalized and treated if necessary, to reduce symptoms. We must not fear it, or there are methods to prevent it, simply accept it as another stage as a person and as a woman.

From the age of 45, early menopause can also occur, which usually occurs between 50 and 55 years.

From 50 Years Old

During the 50s, women begin to suffer from menopause, which is the absence of menstruation for more than 12 months and is due to the permanent cessation of follicular function. Its diagnosis is clinical and retrospective when 12 months have elapsed since the last period without any menstrual bleeding.

Lucas's conception clarifies that "there are no clear guidelines on how to deal with it because each woman has different experiences, but most of the changes in their bodies are related to it."

During this period, the alteration in the distribution of body fat continues. The appearance of the skin in terms of elasticity and hydration worsens, vaginal dryness and other mucous membranes that can cause pain during sexual intercourse are experienced, muscle tone decreases, and muscle damage deteriorates. In addition, bones of the spine, joints, or osteoarthritis problems appear.

"It also increases cardiovascular risk, sleep and memory disorders influenced by the gradual loss of estrogen," explains the specialist, adding that lifestyle changes can cause several mood changes: "during this stage, it is normal to suffer more anxiety, depression and a decrease in mood."

In the fifth decade, the woman may also notice that she loses pubic and axillary hair and undergoes changes in hair and skin or increases in body weight.

Menopause causes, between 50 and 60 years, the woman's skin experiences many alterations. "The decrease in estrogen that occurs at this time in the woman's life leads to a thinning of the skin and dehydration, which causes wrinkles to intensify and 'sagging' of structures.

Acclimatizing the body to the symptoms of menopause by reducing body temperature with light clothing and drinking cold drinks, and exercising regularly to prevent osteoporosis. Proper nutrition, controlled breathing exercises, gynecological exams, and other medical check-ups are also tipping to keep in mind during this stage and during the sixth decade of our life.

The specialist also recalls that the gynaecologist must be present throughout the woman's life, adapting her actions to the different health and reproductive status.

At every stage of the woman, physical changes and psychological changes occur, so that the specialist must be a foothold to ask constantly. "These are vital phases that must be accepted and lived. You don't understand or doubt what you have; you will have your gynecologist solve them.

Process of The Change of Our Body and The State of Well-Being

Our health and well-being have taken priority in our daily lives: when we have free time, outside of work and when we are not occupied with occupations, we like to devote ourselves to activities that are healthy and fun: spending time with friends, playing sports, attending social gatherings, or participating in cultural activities, for example.

But, how do we go about attaining mental and physical well-being that will allow us to enjoy life every day and reach our full potential? We learn about new ways to promote our physical and mental health every day, but much information is still out there, and we may not have as much time as we deserve to familiarize ourselves with our health. Therefore, we are featuring a compilation of the best methods to help you feel physically and mentally healthy.

Break with A Sedentary Lifestyle

It does sound a bit cliché, but our way of life is exceptionally sedentary. At times we find ourselves suffering from the stagnation that could lead to depression because we are not taking advantage of our bodies and our surroundings (or, without going too far, procrastinate and waste our free time, making us feel that we do not give up or take advantage of the time we have been given). Getting out into the world is an excellent way to escape this vicious cycle. This simple action could mean a considerable change in our mental state, especially for those who make it happen physically (something that always produces a feeling of health that raises our mood). Make sure you spend some time outside every day. If you spend this much time exercising in the fresh air each day, you should be able to smell the difference in your skin and hair in a few weeks. Walking is one of the healthiest exercises, and it burns the same calories as running, but it requires more effort because we walk faster. Relax and clear the mind.

Try New Things

This may sound like an exaggeration, but every day of our lives, we have the opportunity to experience new things. It is common for travelers to participate in cultural activities that enrich their travel experience. There are activities like watching plays, attending concerts and participating in cultural fairs where one can meet and learn about other cultures, explore different cultural movements of one's own country, and discover new ones.

Chapter 27.Overcoming the "Down" Moments in Intermittent Fasting

It really doesn't matter whether you are a newbie to intermittent fasting or you've been at it for a while. Each day you struggle to the finishing post, to the small window of time when you can eat, but it seems that everywhere you look, people are eating delicious meals and sipping on full-fat flavored coffees. You find yourself resenting them while you sit and sip on a black coffee or a bottle of water, counting down the minutes and hours until you can eat again. Is that you? Most people who do intermittent fasting go through exactly the same thing, but there is one way to get over it: to change your mindset and build up good healthy habits.

Many people who have tried dieting find themselves in a diet mindset — you are either on one or you aren't. You are either being good or you are cheating on your diet. And, it follows that you are either losing weight or gaining it.

The same goes for intermittent fasting. You will, without a doubt, go at it with the same mindset – you'll reach your goal, and then you'll work out how to maintain it. The biggest problem is that too many people see intermittent fasting as a temporary fix to the temporary problem of weight gain. The actual problem is in mindset. You must learn to see intermittent fasting as a permanent way of life, and the only way to fix your mindset is to change it permanently. You need to shed the diet mindset, and then you will start to see the results you want. You are no longer on a diet. There is no longer a point at which you stop. This is for life, and the sooner you realize that, the easier it will become.

Now, this is the most important part of all. You will find yourself in another mindset – the 'can't' mindset. I can't eat until 6 pm. I can't eat when everyone else is eating. I can't add cream and sugar to my coffee. Instead of focusing on enjoying your lifestyle, you will be focusing on what you see as deprivation. Instead of thinking about what you can do, you constantly think about what you can't do.

This is the mindset you need to shake off quickly because, until you do, you can't even enjoy intermittent fasting, and, believe me, it is an enjoyable lifestyle.

Instead of telling yourself that you deserve to eat when everyone else is, you need to tell yourself that you deserve your health and you deserve to lose weight more. Make that change, and you'll find yourself cooking for your family without even thinking about whether you can eat or not.

How do you conquer the 'can't' mindset? How easy is it? Some people would find it easier than others, but the one thing you can do is read the advantages of intermittent fasting over and over again. Weight loss may be your goal, but intermittent fasting is about so much more. It's about cleansing your body and slowing the aging process. It's about improving your health and having more energy. It's about rediscovering yourself, the person that you are meant to be.

You need to understand that it has nothing to do with not being able to eat when you want; it's all about choosing not to. It's about choosing to understand that your body doesn't need that much food. It's about realizing that your body will benefit from consuming the right foods while still allowing it to rest and heal daily. It's all about seeing the fat melt away with only one quick lifestyle adjustment. Where's the hardship in that? Where's the deprivation when you find yourself fitting into clothes you never thought you'd ever be able to wear again?

So, are you ready to make a huge change in your life? Change your mindset, and you'll be happier and healthier than you ever knew. And this all leads to something else — a change in your eating habits.

Because you can only eat during a certain window of time, you'll want to make the most of it. By feeding your body healthy, nutritious, and delicious foods, you won't want to go back to eating junk. Sure, you can 'treat' yourself occasionally, but I promise you this — after a while on intermittent fasting, you won't want those treats once your body gets used to eating a healthier diet.

One more thing you need to understand — this won't happen overnight. You have to work at changing both your mindset and your habits, so be patient and give yourself time.

Chapter 28.Combining Intermittent Fasting with Other Diets

Now let's start exploring what to eat. As we start looking into what we eat, it's important to talk about the possibility of "supercharging" your fast by adding a diet. Before we get into the different types of diets you can combine with the 16/8 method of intermittent fasting. It's important to make sure you understand the goals. We'll also talk about the benefits and risks and when to combine the two. Before you consider adding a diet to your fast, please make sure you talk to a doctor, especially if you have a medical condition you're concerned about.

Intermittent fasting isn't a diet. It doesn't require any changes to the type of food you eat, though that's recommended if you want to reap the most benefits. While most people will simply eat well-balanced, nutritious meals, you may want to add a diet if you have a very specific goal. If you are already dieting and want to add intermittent fasting to your eating plan, that's great! Just keep in mind that fasting will add some additional stress to your body, and it won't be compatible with some diets. Some examples of diets that don't work with intermittent fasting are low-calorie diets, diets that only focus on one or two food items, and any diet marketed as a cleanse.

Very low-calorie diets (like 800 calories a day) and fasting don't mix for some pretty obvious reasons. If you're not getting enough calories and not eating frequently, you've created a dangerous recipe. Your body won't do well with such a restriction, and you'll likely be malnourished and go into "starvation mode," where your body starts slowing down your metabolism. So, you won't see any results with this type of diet.

. Fasting requires you to have enough energy from your food to make sure you're functioning well during your day, but if your food choice is only, say, cabbage soup, you're not going to get the right nutrients to power your day. You'll end up feeling weak, faint, or nauseous. It's also likely that remaining on such a diet will cause you to have some malnourishment, as there is no way you're getting enough nutrition from cabbage soup alone.

Finally, diets that claim to be "cleansing" diets won't really work with fasting. This is because most cleansing diets are liquid-based and don't really offer nutrition. You will feel incredibly hungry on these cleanses while also fasting. Cleanses aren't necessary since your body can handle itself. So instead, choose diets that are nutritious, healthy, and will provide your body with enough energy to get through your fasting period.

Two diets do work well with intermittent fasting and have some scientific research to back them up. These two diets are the keto diet and some basic calorie restriction. Some people do more calorie restrictions than the unplanned version that naturally comes with fasting but still eat more than 1,200 calories a day. Whichever way you choose, please proceed with caution. You don't want to end up in a state where you are shaking and have a foggy mind. Let's look at these two types of diets.

Keto

The keto diet can help people lose weight, but did you also know that it has been historically used to reduce epilepsy? The keto diet can also help with several diseases like diabetes, skin issues, heart disease, and cancer (Paoli et al., 2013). There is a lot of research to back up these claims. It uses food as medicine to help heal your body. For people who have epilepsy, eating very low-carb foods every day can help ease symptoms and even replace medications. Of course, please just don't throw your meds out. Talk to your doctor first.

So, the keto diet has a lot of positives, but why does it work? You reduce your carbohydrates and increase your healthy fats and proteins in the keto diet. Your carbs are greatly reduced. It's not just a low-carb diet but a very-low-carb diet. Instead of eating carbs, you're eating more healthy fats. In this state, your body starts burning a lot of your stored fat instead of taking energy from carbs (that you're no longer eating). This may sound familiar since intermittent fasting does a very similar thing. It also puts your body into a state of using your stores of fat during the fasting period rather than using what you recently ate. Therefore, the keto diet and intermittent fasting can work together so well.

. The body uses ketones to fuel itself instead of relying on glucose, which is what we get out of carbs and sugary foods. The science behind ketosis and reaching that state is beyond this book's purpose. So, to get to the point, to follow the keto diet, you need to reach the stage of ketosis. To reach this metabolic state, you must consume less than 50 grams of carbohydrates a day. That is not a lot at all. This is about 5% of your daily nutrition in comparison to our normal carb intake, which is well over 50% of our daily nutrition. So, it can be a little difficult to start the process of reducing carbs in such a drastic way.

Ketosis shouldn't be confused with ketoacidosis. Ketosis is healthy. Ketoacidosis is not. Ketoacidosis can affect someone with uncontrollable diabetes or uncontrollable alcohol consumption. It is the result of very high blood sugar levels that then turn your normal, benign blood into something that is highly acidic. Acid running through your veins is not healthy. If left untreated, ketoacidosis is deadly.

So, the keto diet's purpose is to get you into the state of ketosis. It's in this state that you'll burn your fat stores and lose weight. You'll also reap the other benefits of ketosis. Because you are losing your fat stores, you don't have to count your calories. You'll still eat large portions, just without the carbs. The absence of carbs means that you won't be converting them into stores of fat for later energy. You'll be replacing the carbs with higher amounts of healthy fats and proteins. This means you'll feel fuller longer, and eating this way will suppress some of your appetite and cravings.

Combining fasting with the keto diet can help you shed more weight and reach ketosis faster than doing the keto diet alone. This is because fasting already primes your body to burn more fat instead of requiring carbs for an energy source. Again, this is something closely connected to the keto diet.

So, combining keto and intermittent fasting could lead to better glucose levels, lower insulin levels, and better weight loss. Combining calorie restriction with intermittent fasting can result in weight loss, better physiological health, and better aging.

This will help you plan the appropriate steps and better understand the risks associated with combining.

Some people may find it difficult to start and maintain the keto diet. Since it's a restrictive diet, a lot of people's favorite foods may not fit into the diet. This can cause some people to struggle. A way to go about reducing this discomfort is to make the change slowly. Just like we do for intermittent fasting, it takes a couple of weeks to make your changes so that it's not such a huge jarring change. This may make it easier to follow the keto diet.

When first starting keto, many people feel some physiological changes that aren't positive, including poor sleep, a feeling of fogginess, and digestive issues. It can also cause some difficulty with your energy levels, including when you exercise. So you'll need to be prepared for any of these feelings, and they'll pass after a couple of weeks during the following keto.

There is an additional risk that you may lose some muscle when dieting with keto or doing calorie restrictions. This is a risk that comes with any diet. If you're not getting enough protein or nutrients, your body will start taking energy from your muscles instead of your fats. To reduce this risk, make sure that you are eating enough and that it is well-balanced food. Don't just eat junk and expect your body to be okay with it. You'll lose more muscle like that.

With calorie restriction, there are risks like restricting your calories too much. If you do this while on a fast, your body will go into starvation mode, and you won't lose any weight. In fact, each time you eat, your body will start storing energy to prepare for the "starvation" period. Another risk is that you won't eat enough high-quality meals. This can lead to hunger during your fasting window. This isn't ideal, obviously. So, to combat this, make sure you eat well-balanced meals as part of your calorie restriction. It's important to get enough nutrition, so don't base all your food around one food group only.

Chapter 29.Intermittent Fasting Success Stories

If you're still unsure, look at those who have gone before you. These stories are from real women who have lost weight using IF. Most people who try this way of eating are very happy with their results. Some people are mad because they cannot lose weight rapidly or because they have no results because they eat mountains of food in their eating windows. The ones who do it right are inspirational successes.

Amanda's Fasting Story (54 Years Old-Manager Software Development)

I'm not sure how I first became aware of IF. Probably some celebrity-inspired me. Generally, I hate diets, and I would never have undergone this type of nutritional restriction. I believe in enjoying life and eating when you want to. But I had several health problems, including being overweight. I was actually thirty pounds overweight. Plus, my prior attempts to not eat after 6 o'clock didn't work at all, but I have lost all thirty pounds using IF.

I read that you should go for 10 to 20 hours without eating. So, I chose to go 16 hours without eating as a nice middle ground. Thus, I eat at 5 pm and then go to bed and have breakfast at eight. Obviously, it's worked for me.

But I will tell you what was so hard. The hard part was not eating a nighttime meal. I had to get over that and just sip hot chicory tea. That's a lifesaver, by the way. I love chicory tea. I miss milk, but I use tea and water to fill the 15-16 fasting hours. I keep myself busy and sleep like a baby. It helped me get over the need to snack before bed. Now I enjoy my meals so much more. They are not a routine or chore to fix but a pleasure that I look forward to.

I loved how adjustable it is too. One time I had a late office dinner. Easy enough, I just switched breakfast to be at 11 am. It works seamlessly with your schedule. Just keep on top of the hours, and you're good.

During my first month, I dropped ten pounds. Whoohoo! It showed right away. People kept giving me compliments. I didn't mean for these awesome results; they just happened. I didn't have any food restrictions, and I didn't hate my life. I just had to watch when I ate. That's all.

And my stomach has decreased in inches. I can fit old dresses again! I eat smaller portions as a result. The minute I get full, I don't want to eat anymore. I eat in the morning, but I usually don't want to; I chew to get my calories. I have lost edema in most of my body, and my blood pressure is normal. I sleep better because of the chicory, too. I have no more constipation or stomach pain. I recommend this approach to everyone, and I think everyone should adhere to it as much as possible. It's a great program that works with your body.

Rose' Fasting Story (58 Years Old – System Architects)

I found out about the 16:8 fasting system by accident, and I researched it thoroughly. I also asked friends and acquaintances. They had all loved it. As a result, I decided to try it and report back on my results.

I've been following this strategy for three weeks now. I've lost ten pounds already. I sprint for 16 hours before eating for eight. The fasting starts after I eat dinner and lasts for 16 hours until I have breakfast. Generally, I eat at 8 pm and then again at noon. I just adjust the times if I eat earlier or later. Anyone can do it because it is so easy. I don't have any dietary restrictions, but I do now consume more protein. After that, my body simply rests and cleanses for the next 16 hours.

It was initially very challenging. Going to work without breakfast felt like committing some kind of sin because I was taught to believe that breakfast is the most important meal of the day. My whole life, I would eat a big breakfast of cereal, boiled eggs, sandwiches, and even a smoothie. Giving it up made me feel like something was wrong. My schedule was all out-of-whack for a few days, and I was incredibly hungry by lunchtime. By the end of a week, though, that all passed. I began to feel lighter and did not look at the clock waiting for noon.

You don't have to skip breakfast, by the way. That's just what I did. You can eat in the morning and eat dinner earlier. If you need your morning meal, do it. That's what is great about this system; you can make it work for you. I can honestly say that I don't miss breakfast much, though.

You are not obligated to give up any of your favorite foods. You're always allowed to enjoy your favorite dessert. I love chocolate, so I eat that during my window. What diet allows you to do that? Uh, this one! But this plan isn't really a diet, just a power system. I feel light, and I'm losing fat, not muscle mass. Don't torture yourself with fad diets that don't work; use this power system and enjoy the results. Intermitting fasting is really just a simple lifestyle change you can fit into your daily life.

Ellice's Fasting Story (55 Years Old – Finance Manager)

I had pretty much given up on remission from rheumatoid arthritis after giving birth. I was on the verge of despair, both physically and mentally. My quality of life was so low. Drug treatments don't work well for me, and my family has a long history of Type 1

Diabetes. I knew that I would develop diabetes because of my pancreas's sudden jumps. I knew something wasn't right because I'd break out in cold sweats and feel really weak before eating. I was at a loss for what to do, and my choices appeared to be limited.

But on some baby board, I found some women raving about IF. Well, why not try it? Nothing else was working.

I started experimenting with it. It wasn't so bad. I have started going longer times with my fasts. Recently, I made it 36 hours! After starting this practice, I noticed that I felt way better in the mornings. Usually, I hurt the worst in my joints at this time, so the pain was subsiding. One day about a week in, I woke up feeling light, like my depression had lifted. Then I realized that I hadn't eaten since 4 pm the day before. I was distracted and forgot supper. I guess that happens, but it showed me that I don't need three meals a day, as they say.

Maybe my body couldn't spare as much for autoimmune processes if I didn't have so much protein in my system from dinner. Or maybe if my organs were resting and not moving so much with digestion, they did not make so many extra movements and enzymes. Maybe my body was getting rid of toxins. Perhaps this approach was the secret to getting well from my RA.

So now I do IF, and I restrict my solid food, but I drink all the water I want. Over three months, my condition has improved a lot; I'm a lot more flexible, and I have no more reflux esophagitis!

The only bad thing is that I have to stick with this for life. I broke my regimen once, and my symptoms flared up like clockwork. This plan will be for life. But it's not so bad. It is super easy to follow. The elders knew something when they said not to eat after 6!

Chapter 30.New Healthy Habits

Once you get started with intermittent fasting, you will soon notice a natural tendency towards a more generally healthy lifestyle. This is a quite common virtuous circle: you start with a single healthy choice; this makes you feel better, feeling better gives you the energy to go on with more healthy choices, in a snowball effect of wellness.

You will naturally know and feel what healthy changes you'll need to put into your life, and this will probably concern your body's health and mind and spirit. For instance, once I kept experiencing increased clarity, I naturally felt the desire to read more books and scheduled a daily "me-time" of 45 minutes, door closed, and phone off.

So, now we are going to look at some aspects you should consider as a general lifestyle background for your intermittent fasting path; still, this is just some advice. Please listen to yourself and be ready to embrace your body, mind, and spirit suggestions.

Moderate, If You Don't Want to Get Rid of, Alcohol

Intermittent fasting has been shown to diminish inflammation in your body.

In any case, alcohol may aggravate inflammation, limiting the benefits of this diet.

Chronic inflammation may advance different diseases, for example, heart disease, type 2 diabetes, and certain malignancies.

Research shows that inflammation from excessive drinking may prompt intestinal disorder, bacterial overgrowth, and anomalies in intestinal microorganisms.

High alcohol intake can likewise strain your liver, diminishing its capacity to sift through possibly damaging elements.

Together, these consequences for your intestine and liver may advance inflammation all through your body, which can cause organ harm over time.

Over the top alcohol intake can cause far-reaching inflammation in your body, slowing if not stopping the effects of intermittent fasting and conceivably prompting infections.

Also, consider that drinking alcohol can break your fast.

During a fast, you should avoid all foods and drinks for a certain amount of time.

In particular, intermittent fasting is intended to advance hormonal and physical changes —for example, fat consumption and cell repair— that may benefit your health.

As alcohol contains calories, any amount of it during a fasting period will break your fast. It is also perfectly acceptable to drink in moderation during your eating periods.

During fasting periods, your body starts cell repair processes like autophagy, in which old, harmed proteins are expelled from cells to produce more effective, healthier cells.

This process may diminish your danger of malignancy, distances the issues of aging effects, and at any rate, somewhat clarifies why calorie limitation has been shown to expand life expectancy.

Ongoing animal studies showing that constant alcohol intake may hinder autophagy in the liver and fat tissue.

Picking Better Alcohol Choices

As alcohol breaks your fast whenever expended during a fasting period, it is recommended to just drink during your planned eating periods. You should likewise hold your intake under tight restraints. Moderate alcohol consumption is characterized as close to one drink a day for women and close to two a day for men.

While intermittent fasting does not have exacting food and drink intake standards, some alcohol habits are healthier than others and more averse to hindering your dietary routine.

To restrict your sugar and calorie intake, avoid cocktails and prefer wines. It is ideal to drink alcohol moderately and only during your eating windows during intermittent fasting.

The Unhindered Eating Trap

Anyone who has ever changed their diet to get a health benefit or a healthy weight realizes that you begin to desire foods that you are recommended not to eat. Truth be told, a study published in 2017 affirmed that an increased drive to eat is a key factor during a weight loss journey.

Nevertheless, this test is explicitly restricted to an intermittent fasting plan. Food limitation just happens during certain restricted hours, and on the non-fasting hours or days of the plan, you can eat anything you desire for the most part.

Obviously, keeping on with unhealthy foods may not be the healthiest way to pick up benefits from intermittent fasting; however, removing them during specific days restricts your overall intake and may, in the end, give benefits anyway.

Don't Stop Working Out

Or start doing it if you didn't.

You don't need to be an athlete, but you can't afford a sedentary lifestyle. Some people may think that they should save energy and rest a lot since they are fasting. Well, that's not exactly like this. You should exercise as much as you can (that could be a little for you, but still), just taking some care.

You should choose whether you want to work out while fasting or after eating. On the chance that you stick to the early afternoon to 8 P.M. eating plan, this mainly comes down to whether you usually work out in the first part of the day or in the evening. Remember that you can change your timetable to your necessities. If you want to work out toward the beginning of the day after eating, you can change your fasting and eating periods to do it.

Training During Fasting

Training in a fasted state requires a few supplements to keep your body in an anabolic state. The body utilizes amino acids for energy if you are training without a pre-exercise meal. Therefore, your supplements for fast ought to include glutamine and branched-chain amino acid (BCAA) supplements.

Following the early afternoon to 8 P.M. feeding plan, you fast from 8 P.M. until around noon. So, take your glutamine and BCAA enhancements, and then do your workout. Depending on how long your workout will last, this will set your post-exercise meal around the early afternoon.

What number of meals you decide to have during your starting period is up to you; however, remember that eating less as often as possible can hold your yearning within proper limits and support your body's capacity to build muscle.

Training During Feeding Period

On the chance that you like to work out after eating, you can plan your exercise to fall in the afternoon (early around 1 pm, or toward the evening, around 5 pm). On the other hand, if your workout session is, for the most part, in the late afternoon, have your pre-training meal around the early afternoon, work out, and afterwards have your other meals.

For an evening session, have your first meal around early afternoon and your pre-exercise meal around 4 P.M. If you may want to have a post-training meal one hour after working out, you can do that.

Adjusting Your Calorie Intake

The main principles of intermittent fasting include a few directions on when and how to get your calories and macronutrients.

If you train while fasting, the calorie check of your BCAA supplement should be calculated toward your complete calories of the day, even though it does not end your fasting period. For example, people on intermittent fasting plans normally distribute fifty calories for their fasting period to take into account things like supplements or refreshments. This implies you can, in any case, take cream and sugar in your espresso or tea, regardless of whether or not it is during your fasting period.

If you're going to eat a pre-workout meal, it's best to keep it light. For a total of 400-500 calories, your meal should include a protein source such as poultry or fish and some carbohydrates. This will provide you with the protein and complex carbohydrates that are commonly recommended for pre-workout meals. If you do eat a pre-exercise meal, the BCAA supplements prescribed for fasting exercises are most likely redundant, but you might need to take them in any case since having an overflow of BCAAs may now be helpful anyway.

Your post-training meal is the best time to take a large portion of your sugars and calories. About a big part of your total calories for the day ought to be eaten during your post-training meal.

Conclusion

Intermittent fasting for women over 50 is a highly successful weight-loss strategy because it has many health benefits. In chronically depressed individuals, intermittent fasting has improved mood and concentration, increased serotonin and dopamine levels, reduced inflammation in brain tissue and blood vessel walls, and reduced anxiety.

According to studies, women over 50 who fasted for 24 hours a week saw a major reduction in inflammation in their blood vessels, brain, and heart. When compared to people who didn't fast, people who followed an intermittent fasting diet plan had a 40% lower level of inflammation in their blood vessels and a 50% lower level of inflammatory markers (specifically C-reactive Protein) in their blood than those who did not participate in any fasting program.

Other studies found that highly active women over 50 had a significant drop in inflammation levels when they fasted for just 6 hours per week (less than one full day per week). Those who followed a fasting diet plan lowered their inflammatory markers by 20% and their C-reactive Protein marker by 32%!

This is fantastic news because high levels of inflammation are a known trigger of things like heart disease, cancer, and other age-related diseases. If you can reduce your inflammatory markers through dieting alone, without having to resort to expensive prescription drugs or invasive medical procedures, it would be foolish not to do so. In addition, intermittent fasting has been shown to help people reach both their physical health goals as well as psychological goals.

Intermittent fasting for women over 50 can also benefit your social life and increase your overall happiness. Those who fasted regularly reported feeling less anxiety and more focus throughout the day as compared to those who were not involved in any intermittent fasting program. This result was likely influenced by elevated levels of natural endorphins (happy hormones) that are created during a fast.

But intermittent fasting isn't just a dieting method that you can use to reach your physical or psychological goals; it is also an effective way to prevent disease in older women. Studies have shown that people who follow an intermittent fasting program live longer than those who don't participate, but this effect is most pronounced in overweight individuals. For example, women who followed a fasting diet plan had a 35% lower risk of death than those who did not. In addition, intermittent fasting reduces the risk of diseases like diabetes, cardiac disease, and cancer by up to 20% in overweight people.

So, how can women over 50 enjoy the benefits of intermittent fasting? If you're over the age of 51, skip breakfast and fast for 16 hours between lunch and dinner. Miss breakfast and fast until lunchtime if you're under 51 years old. The only way to do this is to rise before your alarm goes off. You can still eat dinner that night, but you won't be eating lunch. Just remember to include at least 16 hours of fasting time (plus an hour or two for sleeping) between dinner and breakfast each day. This is intermittent fasting for women over 50 at its simplest.

Chapter 31. Vegetarian Intermittent Fasting Recipes

1.   Vegan Tofu Barbeque

Have you ever made tofu in a crockpot? If not, try this weekend's tofu barbecue, which is full of flavor and homemade sauce. It is a slow cooker recipe that you can easily make at any time. Just put all the ingredients in your crockpot in the morning and let it soak in all the flavors slowly. By the time you come back home, you will have a delicious sweet and savory dish ready to be served. Combine it with rice or whole grains of your choice for a complete meal.

Time: 5 hours 5 minutes

Serving Size: 4–6 servings

Prep Time: 5 minutes

Cook Time: 5 hours

Nutritional Facts/Info:

Calories	213 kcal
Carbs	24 g
Fat	8 g
Protein	16 g
Fiber	2 g

Ingredients:

- 2 (14 oz) blocks tofu
- 1 1/2 cups ketchup
- 3 tbsp brown sugar
- 1 tbsp apple cider vinegar
- 1/2 tsp garlic powder
- Kosher salt, to taste
- 2 tbsp soy sauce
- 1 tsp red chili flakes
- Black pepper, to taste

Directions:

1. Gather all the ingredients.
2. Press tofu to release all the water.
3. Cut it into bite-sized pieces and combine it with the other ingredients in the slow cooker.
4. Cover it and cook on low heat for at least 5–6 hours.
5. Serve it hot!

2.   Mexican Quinoa

Here is another quick recipe for you. This Mexican quinoa made with black beans and corn is high in protein and makes a perfect dinner recipe for when you are lazy.

Time: 25 minutes

Serving Size: 4 servings

Prep Time: 5 minutes

Cook Time: 20 minutes

Nutritional Facts/Info:

Calories	338 kcal
Carbs	60 g
Fat	9 g
Protein	13 g
Fiber	13 g

Ingredients:

- Quinoa
- 1 red onion
- Black beans
- Frozen corn
- Garlic
- Cumin
- Fresh lime juice
- 2 bell peppers
- Paprika powder
- Vegetable broth
- Diced tomatoes
- Chopped parsley
- Salt and pepper
- Red chili flakes (optional)

Directions:

1. In a large pot, heat some oil and sauté the onion for around 2–3 minutes. Once it becomes translucent, add garlic and bell pepper and cook for 2 more minutes on high heat.
2. Add all the other ingredients except for green onions, parsley, and lime juice.

3. Cover and cook for 20 minutes. Keep checking in between to see if the quinoa is burning or sticking to the base.

4. Once it's done, add lime juice, parsley, and green onions. Season it with salt and pepper, and serve.

3.   Lentil Meatballs

These savory meatballs are rich in healthy ingredients such as lentils, garlic, onion, soy sauce, tomatoes, and more. All these make this a power-packed dish.

Time: 2 hours

Serving Size: 6 servings

Prep Time: 55 minutes

Cook Time: 1 hour 5 minutes

Nutritional Facts/Info:

Calories	312 kcal
Carbs	70 g
Fat	12 g
Protein	18 g
Fiber	11 g

Ingredients:

For the sauce:

- 2 tbsp olive oil
- 28 oz crushed tomatoes
- 4 cloves garlic
- Handful of basil leaves
- Kosher salt

For the meatballs:

- 1 cup rinsed brown lentils
- 3 tbsp olive oil
- 4 oz mushrooms
- 5 cloves garlic
- 2 slices white bread
- 1/3 cup wheat berries
- 1 small yellow onion
- 3 tbsp tomato paste
- 3 tbsp low-sodium soy sauce
- 2 tbsp red wine vinegar
- Kosher salt
- Black pepper

- 4 tsp nutritional yeast
- 1/2 cup fresh parsley leaves

Directions:

1. For the sauce, put the oil and garlic in a saucepan on medium heat. Mix until you get that garlic fragrance. Add tomatoes and water, simmer, and keep the heat medium-low. Add basil leaves and salt and simmer without covering for around 25 minutes.

2. For the meatballs, preheat the oven to 400 degrees Fahrenheit. Put a baking sheet and brush with some oil.

3. Add water to a medium saucepan and bring it to a boil. Add the wheat berries and boil until it turns tender. Drain it and keep it aside.

4. Boil the lentils and then reduce heat to low without covering until the water evaporates. Drain it and let it cool.

5. Heat oil in a skillet. Add onions, garlic, mushrooms, salt, and pepper and cook until light brown. Add tomatoes, vinegar, soy sauce, and yeast, and cook until the water has evaporated. Let it cool.

6. Add the mixture to a food processor with lentils, parsley, and wheat berries. Pulse until it is crumbly.

7. Soak the bread in the water and then mash it. Add the lentil mixture and mix it by hand. Make it into small balls.

8. Place them on a baking sheet about 1 inch apart and bake until they turn golden brown.

9. Serve with the sauce and garnish with some parsley.

4.   Vegan Fettuccine Alfredo

Here is another quick recipe for you. This Mexican quinoa made with black beans and corn is high in protein and makes a perfect dinner recipe for when you are lazy.

Time: 25 minutes

Serving Size: 4 servings

Prep Time: 15 minutes

Cook Time: 10 minutes

Nutritional Facts/Info:

Calories	498 kcal
Carbs	70 g
Fat	19 g
Protein	12 g
Fiber	6 g

Ingredients:

- 8 oz fettuccine pasta
- 2 tbsp flour
- 2 1/4 cups soy milk
- 1/4 cup olive oil
- 3 tbsp thyme
- Salt and black pepper, to taste
- Steamed veggies (optional)

Directions:

1. Fill a medium saucepan halfway with water.
2. Bring it to a boil and add the pasta. Cook until al dente (almost cooked) and drain.
3. For the sauce, heat the oil in a saucepan.
4. Add flour and cook for 2 minutes. Stir constantly until smooth.
5. While stirring, add soy milk and thyme and bring to a simmer. After 4–5 minutes, add salt and pepper.
6. Serve with steamed veggies and fettuccine, and enjoy!

5. Vegetarian Casserole

This bite-ready salad recipe is both filling and easy to make. Packed with a yummy coleslaw mix, this is the perfect everyday breakfast (or lunch) recipe.

Time: 3 hours

Serving Size: 4 servings

Prep Time: 2 hours 15 minutes

Cook Time: 45 minutes

Nutritional Facts/Info:

Calories	323 kcal
Carbs	23 g
Fat	11 g
Protein	18 g
Fiber	1 g

Ingredients:

- 1 14-oz sausage substitute
- 1 1/2 cups milk (any milk)
- 6 eggs
- 1 tbsp onion, chopped
- 4 slices whole-grain bread
- 1 tbsp cooking oil

- 1/2 to 3/4 cup cheddar cheese
- 1 cup spinach (optional)

Directions:

1. In a skillet, heat the oil and sauté the sausage and onions for 5 minutes until it turns light brown.
2. Cover a pan with the sausage substitute.
3. Cut the slices of bread into 1-inch strips and place them across the sausage.
4. Take a bowl and mix into it the eggs and milk. Add the chopped spinach if you want to, and pour the mixture evenly over the bread. Top off with some shredded cheese.
5. Cover it and keep it in the fridge for two hours or until the bread has soaked up the mixture.
6. Preheat oven to 350 degrees Fahrenheit.
7. Bake the casserole for about 35–45 minutes until golden.
8. Cut in pieces and serve hot!

6. Asian Fusion Tacos

Fan of tacos? Then you won't be able t0 resist this Asian-inspired taco recipe made with Asian ingredients and combined with a delicious and creamy topping.

Time: 40 minutes

Serving Size: 4 servings

Prep Time: 15 minutes

Cook Time: 25 minutes

Nutritional Facts/Info:

Calories	350 kcal
Carbs	28 g
Fat	24 g
Protein	6 g
Fiber	4 g

Ingredients:

- 10 tbsp salad dressing
- 6 cups cauliflower florets
- 2 cloves garlic
- 1 tbsp soy sauce
- 2 tsp ground ginger
- 8 soft taco-size flour tortillas
- 1 package (3.5 oz) sliced shiitake mushrooms (or any)

Directions:

1. Preheat the oven to 400 °F. Line your baking sheet with parchment paper.

2. Combine all the ingredients in a bowl. Transfer 1/4 cup of the mixture to a large bowl and save the remaining for drizzling.

3. Add mushrooms and cauliflower to the bigger bowl and mix. Spread on the baking sheet and roast for 25 minutes.

4. Put the vegetables on the taco shells, then drizzle with the sauce. Garnish with chopped cilantro, green onions, and red bell pepper.

7. Acapulco Slaw

This bite-ready salad recipe is both filling and easy to make. Packed with a yummy coleslaw mix, this is the perfect everyday breakfast (or lunch) recipe.

Time: 15 minutes

Serving Size: 4 servings

Prep Time: 15 minutes

Cook Time: 0 minutes

Nutritional Facts/Info:

Calories	510 kcal
Carbs	21 g
Fat	4 g
Protein	6 g
Fiber	6 g

Ingredients:

- 1 cup mayonnaise
- 2 tbsp sugar
- 2 tbsp lime juice
- 1 bag (16 oz) coleslaw mix
- 1 medium jalapeno pepper
- 2 tbsp chopped cilantro
- 1 tbsp cumin seeds, toasted
- 1/2 tsp salt
- 1/4 tsp black pepper

Directions:

1. In a large bowl, combine all the ingredients. Refrigerate the mixture.

2. When serving, sprinkle some cheese and enjoy!

8. Vegetarian Shepherd's Pie

This vegetarian shepherd's pie, crafted with green peas, sauce, and corn, is a filling, satisfying, and flavorful main dish that's suitable for vegetarians, vegans, and non-vegetarians alike.

Time: 55 minutes

Serving Size: 4 servings

Prep Time: 15 minutes

Cook Time: 40 minutes

Nutritional Facts/Info:

Calories	486 kcal
Carbs	72 g
Fat	12 g
Protein	27 g
Fiber	13 g

Ingredients:

- 4 medium potatoes, chopped
- 1 medium onion, diced
- 2 tbsp margarine
- 1/4 cup soy milk (or any milk)
- 1/2 cup green peas
- 1/2 cup corn
- 1 1/4 cups vegetarian gravy
- 1 tbsp vegetable oil
- 1 1/2 cups vegetarian meat substitute
- 1/2 teaspoon garlic powder
- Cayenne pepper
- Salt and black pepper, to taste

Directions:

1. Preheat oven to 350 degrees Fahrenheit.

2. Boil the potatoes until soft. Mash with the milk and margarine. Add salt and pepper.

3. Sauté the onion until tender.

4. In a bowl, add the onions, beef substitute, gravy, garlic powder, peas, corn, and cayenne pepper. Pour into a baking dish.

5. Spread the potatoes over the mixture.

6. Bake for 30–40 minutes until thoroughly cooked.

9. Oats Veggie Tots

It's a new level of tater tots. You can't go wrong with this recipe because it's full of vegetables such as potatoes and zucchini! With this recipe, you can easily get more veggies and nutrients into your diet. With so many veggies, they make for the perfect healthy snack

Time: 1 hour 10 minutes

Serving Size: 37 tots

Prep Time: 10 minutes

Cook Time: 1 hour

Nutritional Facts/Info:

Calories	666 kcal
Carbs	36.4 g
Fat	18.5 g
Protein	9.1 g
Fiber	1.3 g

Ingredients:

- 1 large zucchini
- 1/2 small cauliflower
- 1 medium carrot, peeled
- 1 medium potato, peeled
- 1 tsp salt
- 2 flax eggs
- 1/2 medium diced onion
- 1/3 cup breadcrumbs
- 2 cloves garlic, finely minced
- 1/3 cup parmesan cheese
- Black pepper, to taste
- 1/4 cup finely chopped parsley

Directions:

1. Grate the zucchini, cauliflower, potato, and carrot. Transfer to a bowl and mix, and add salt. Allow the vegetables to sit for 20 minutes to draw out the moisture.

2. Prepare the flax egg by mixing together two tablespoons of flaxseed meal and six tablespoons of water. Let it sit.

3. Preheat the oven to 400 °F. Line a baking sheet with parchment paper.

4. Transfer the vegetables to a clean kitchen towel. Strain out any liquid from the vegetables.

5. Place them into the bowl and add the flax eggs, parmesan, white onion, parsley, garlic, breadcrumbs, pepper, and salt. Mix well.

6. Take out one tablespoon and make a tater tot shape. Do the same with the rest of the mixture.

7. Put on the baking sheet and into the oven for 25–30 minutes or until golden brown, flipping halfway through.

8. Let it cool and serve with the sauce of your choice. Enjoy!

10. Pasta Salad

Pasta and salad? That doesn't sound so good, but the recipe is indeed delicious! Plus, it has fewer ingredients and requires minimal cooking and prepping time.

Time: 18 minutes

Serving Size: 8 servings

Prep Time: 10 minutes

Cook Time: 8 minutes

Nutritional Facts/Info:

Calories	300 kcal
Carbs	38 g
Fat	16 g
Protein	5 g
Fiber	1 g

Ingredients:

- 1 box spaghetti
- 3 cups Napa cabbage
- 2 tbsp vinegar
- 2 tbsp soy sauce
- 2 tsp toasted sesame oil
- ¾ cup dressing
- 1 cup shredded carrots
- 1/2 cup chopped cilantro

Directions:

1. Cook spaghetti, drain, and rinse with cold water.

2. Mix the dressing, vinegar, soy sauce, and sesame oil in a bowl. Gently add the spaghetti and the rest of the ingredients. Cover and refrigerate for at least one hour.

3. Season with some parsley and serve.

11. Tofu and Spinach Scramble

This recipe is ideal for vegans who are looking for an omelet-ish dish for breakfast. Crumbled tofu is sautéed with vegetables to imitate scrambled eggs. You will not even notice that you're not actually eating eggs!

Time: 15 minutes

Serving Size: 2 to 4 servings

Prep Time: 5 minutes

Cook Time: 10 minutes

Nutritional Facts/Info:

Calories	209 kcal
Carbs	12 g
Fat	13 g
Protein	16 g
Fiber	5 g

Ingredients:

- 2 tbsp olive oil
- 1 pound tofu, pressed
- 3/4 cup sliced mushrooms
- 2 medium tomatoes, chopped
- 1 (10 oz) bunch spinach, rinsed
- 2 garlic cloves, minced
- 1/4 tsp ground turmeric
- 1/2 tsp soy sauce
- 1 tsp lemon juice
- Salt and pepper, to taste

Directions:

1. Heat the oil in a pan and sauté the garlic, mushrooms, and tomatoes over medium heat for around 2–3 minutes.

2. Reduce the heat to low and add the crumbled tofu, turmeric, spinach, soy sauce, and lemon juice. Cover and cook for 5–7 minutes.

3. Season with salt and pepper.

12. Black Beans with Lime Rice

This lime rice recipe made with black beans, onions, and corn and simmered in a flavorful broth is truly undeniable. The best part? It's ready in less than 30 minutes.

Time: 30 minutes

Serving Size: 4 servings

Prep Time: 10 minutes

Cook Time: 20 minutes

Nutritional Facts/Info:

Calories	267 kcal
Carbs	15 g
Fat	10 g
Protein	8 g
Fiber	5 g

Ingredients:

For the beans:

- 2 (15 oz) cans black beans, drained and rinsed
- 2 cups vegetable broth
- 1 small red onion, chopped
- 2/3 cup water
- 2/3 cup corn
- 2 garlic cloves, minced
- 1 tsp Italian seasoning
- 1 tsp cumin
- 1 tsp onion powder
- 1/2 tsp paprika
- 1/2 tsp garlic powder
- 1/2 tsp chili powder
- Salt, to taste
- Cayenne pepper to taste

For the rice:

- 2 cups brown rice
- Lime juice

Directions:

Rice:

1. Cook the rice.

2. Once it's fully cooked, squeeze lime juice and mix.

Beans:

3. In a saucepan, sauté the garlic and onion in 1 tablespoon broth (or more) for 5–7 minutes until it is translucent.

4. Add in the seasonings and sauté for a minute.

5. Add the remaining broth, beans, corn, and water to the saucepan. Cover and simmer for 15 minutes.

6. Add the rice and the beans to a bowl. Serve with some lime wedges, cilantro, and tortilla chips.

13. White Bean Salad

Trying to find a recipe for the best white bean salad? This vegetarian dish is quick and easy to make, and it goes well with just about anything. This simple bean salad can be made with any variety of white beans.

Time: 10 minutes

Serving Size: 4–6 servings

Prep Time: 10 minutes

Cook Time: 0 minutes

Nutritional Facts/Info:

Calories	586 kcal
Carbs	100 g
Fat	7 g
Protein	33 g
Fiber	29 g

Ingredients:

- 2 (15-ounce) cans white beans
- 1/2 cup fresh parsley, chopped
- 2 large tomatoes, diced
- 1/3 cup sliced black olives
- 2 tbsp red wine vinegar
- 1/2 lemon, juiced
- 3 cloves garlic, minced
- 1 red onion, minced
- 2 tbsp olive oil
- Salt and pepper, to taste

Directions:

1. Saute the beans, onion, garlic, and parsley in olive oil for a minute or until fragrant.
2. Transfer to a large bowl.
3. Add the black olives, vinegar, tomatoes, and lemon juice and toss to mix. Add remaining ingredients.
4. Serve warm as it is, or chill before serving.

14. Lentil Soup

When it comes to cooking, lentil soup should be a staple in every kitchen. Lentils are easy to find in most supermarkets, are packed with protein, are good for you, and are very inexpensive. Besides, they are so versatile that you can make this recipe as per your own style with your choice of ingredients.

Time: 55 minutes

Serving Size: 4 servings

Prep Time: 5 minutes

Cook Time: 50 minutes

Nutritional Facts/Info:

Calories	100 kcal
Carbs	17 g
Fat	2 g
Protein	5 g
Fiber	5 g

Ingredients:

- 1 cup dried brown lentils
- 1 onion, diced
- 1 carrot, sliced
- 1 tsp vegetable oil
- 1/4 tsp dried thyme
- 4 cups vegetable broth
- 2 bay leaves
- Salt, to taste
- Ground black pepper, to taste
- 2 tsp lemon juice, optional

Directions:

1. In a pot or pan, sauté the carrots and onion in oil for 3–5 minutes, or until the onions turn translucent.
2. Add the lentils, thyme, bay leaves, broth, salt, and black pepper.
3. Reduce heat to a simmer. Cover and cook until soft, around 45 minutes.
4. Remove the bay leaves and add some lemon juice. Serve warm.

15. Vegetarian Pad Thai

Making vegetarian Pad Thai from scratch is much simpler than you think. Vegan and vegetarian Thai food fans will love this recipe because it doesn't include any meat. Pad Thai's distinctive flavor comes from the tamarind-chili sauce, which is made from scratch and has a unique balance of sweet, savory, and spice.

Time: 31 minutes

Serving Size: 2 servings

Prep Time: 15 minutes

Cook Time: 16 minutes

Nutritional Facts/Info:

Calories	1010 kcal
Carbs	133 g
Fat	42 g
Protein	28 g
Fiber	8 g

Ingredients:

- 8 ounces dried rice noodles

For the sauce:

- 3 tbsp brown sugar
- 1/2 to 1 tsp chili sauce
- 2 1/4 tsp tamarind paste
- 1/4 cup vegetable stock
- 3 1/2 tbsp soy sauce
- 1/8 to 3/4 tsp chili flakes

For the stir-fry:

- 3 to 4 tbsp coconut oil or peanut oil
- 3 to 4 heads baby bok choy
- 2 to 3 tbsp vegetable stock
- 4 cloves garlic, minced
- 3 tbsp diced onion
- 2 green onions, sliced
- 1/4 cup chopped cashews or peanuts
- 1/3 cup cilantro
- 2 wedges lime

Directions:

1. Boil some water for the noodles.
2. Cook the noodles for 4-6 minutes until they are firm, but tender. Drain and rinse.
3. Combine the ingredients for the sauce in a cup and stir well. Add more sugar if needed. Set aside.
4. Put a large frying pan over medium-high heat. Put some oil and stir-fry garlic and onion for one minute.
5. Add bok choy and stock to fry the ingredients nicely. Stir-fry for two minutes.
6. Take out the ingredients and add 1/2 tablespoon of the oil to the pan. Add the egg and stir-fry.
7. Add the noodles and one-third of the sauce. Stir-fry everything for around two minutes.

8. Keep moving from medium to high heat and vice versa, depending on whether the noodles are sticking at the bottom.
9. Continue adding sauce while stir-frying for around six more minutes, or until the sauce is completely added and the noodles are soft. If using tofu, add it last with the sauce. It will break and scatter throughout the dish.
10. Turn off the flame and add green onions, bean sprouts, and some of the nuts. Add more soy sauce if needed. If the flavor is 0verpowering, add some lime juice or sugar to balance it.
11. Scoop the noodles onto a platter. Toss the remaining nuts and cilantro. Fresh-cut lime wedges are to be used when eating.

16. Vegan Summer Rolls

These mint and mango rice paper rolls are a light and refreshing summertime meal. It's fresh, healthy, low in calories, and scrumptious all at once. Dip them in a simple peanut sauce, and voila! Your mouth-watering vegan dish is ready.

Time: 20 minutes

Serving Size: 6 servings

Prep Time: 20 minutes

Cook Time: 0 minutes

Nutritional Facts/Info:

Calories	258 kcal
Carbs	33 g
Fat	12 g
Protein	8 g
Fiber	5 g

Ingredients:

For the rice paper rolls:

- 6 sheets rice paper
- 1 - 1 1/2 cups glass noodles
- 3 small carrots
- 1 avocado
- 1 cucumber
- 1 mango
- 6 radishes
- 1 cup fresh mint
- 3 green onion

- 1 cup purple cabbage
- 2-3 cups lettuce

For the sauce:

- 1/4 cup peanut butter
- 1 clove of garlic, minced
- 2 tsp soy sauce
- 3-4 tbsp warm water
- 1/2 sriracha sauce (optional)

Directions:

1. Cut all of the vegetables into thin strips.
2. Once you are done, fill a bowl with some water and dip the rice papers, so they get wet. Don't let them soak, or they will get too soft.
3. Fill the rice papers with the vegetables and wrap them just like a burrito. It's best to make the filling in the center, roll it up, and fold it sideways.
4. For the sauce, add the peanut butter, soy sauce, warm water, garlic, and the sriracha sauce into a bowl.
5. Serve the rolls with the sauce.

17. Avocado Roast with Balsamic Drizzle

This heaven-in-your-mouth recipe combines avocado, heirloom, tomatoes, and balsamic vinegar, which is perfect for a late summer's evening snack or breakfast. The fresh ingredients used in this recipe will make you feel refreshed and energized!

Time: 25 minutes

Serving Size: 1 servings

Prep Time: 10 minutes

Cook Time: 15 minutes

Nutritional Facts/Info:

Calories	534 kcal
Carbs	64 g
Fat	25 g
Protein	10 g
Fiber	9 g

Ingredients:

- 2-3 slices bread
- ½ cup balsamic vinegar
- Olive oil
- 2 small heirloom tomatoes

- ½ an avocado
- ¼ cup fresh basil, chopped
- Ground black pepper
- Sea salt

Directions:

1. In a small pan, heat the balsamic vinegar on medium-high heat until reduced. While continuously whisking, bring the vinegar to a boil. Cook for around 10–15 minutes, or until the balsamic has whittled down by half and coats a spoon and is thick enough to drizzle. Keep checking it constantly as it burns quickly.
2. Toast the bread after drizzling it with olive oil.
3. Put the avocado evenly over the bread and smash it thoroughly.
4. Finish the layering with sliced tomatoes, fresh herbs, and balsamic reduction.
5. Season with black pepper and salt.
6. Serve right away.

18. Vegan Thai Curry

This quick and easy Thai curry is a must-have for Thai food lovers. It contains antioxidant-rich broccoli and cabbage. Turmeric's anti-inflammatory effects make this a healthy one-bowl supper. This recipe contains no oil beyond the coconut milk's natural fats.

Time: 20 minutes

Serving Size: 4 servings

Prep Time: 5 minutes

Cook Time: 15 minutes

Nutritional Facts/Info:

Calories	223 kcal
Carbs	25 g
Fat	13 g
Protein	6 g
Fiber	21 g

Ingredients:

- 1 cup coconut milk
- 2 medium carrots, sliced
- 1 medium potato, chopped
- 1 cup broccoli florets
- 1 cup vegetable broth

- 1/2 head cauliflower florets
- 3 cloves garlic, minced
- 1/2 tsp ground turmeric
- 1 tbsp fresh ginger
- 1 tsp sugar
- 2 tsp curry powder
- 3 tsp chili sauce
- 1/3 tsp salt
- Juice of a lime, optional
- 1/2 cup cilantro, optional

Directions:

1. In a huge pot, add the vegetable broth and coconut milk and stir. Bring it to a simmer.
2. Add in all your cooked veggies and let the mixture simmer for around 2–3 minutes while stirring in between.
3. Add in the sugar, garlic, ginger, turmeric, curry powder, chili sauce, and salt, and mix well.
4. Allow the curry to cook over medium-low flame for 3–5 minutes, or until the texture of the vegetables becomes tender.
5. Taste, and add more seasonings if needed.
6. While serving, squeeze fresh lime juice and a dash of fresh cilantro.

19. Vegan Quiche

This vegan quiche made with asparagus and tomato is a wonderful addition to any brunch. It's savory, delicious, and easy to put together. It's also extremely versatile, so if you don't like asparagus, you can use any type of vegetable. In order to make the crust, you'll need to chill the dough for a half-hour in the refrigerator before you begin. However, the actual time spent preparing is relatively short.

Time: 1 hr 15 minutes

Serving Size: 8 servings

Prep Time: 50 minutes

Cook Time: 25 minutes

Nutritional Facts/Info:

Calories	325 kcal
Carbs	27 g
Fat	21 g
Protein	10 g

Fiber	4 g

Ingredients:

For the Crust:

- 2 cups whole wheat flour
- 3/4 cup butter (vegan)
- 1/3 cup water
- 1/2 tsp salt

For the Filling:

- 14 oz silken tofu
- 1 tsp turmeric
- 10 sun-dried tomatoes
- 10 cherry tomatoes
- 1 pinch black salt
- 2 tbsp olive oil
- 1 tbsp cornstarch
- 7 oz smoked tofu
- 14 oz green asparagus
- 2 green onions rings
- 1 1/2 tbsp herbs

Directions:

1. For the dough, take a bowl and add all the ingredients. Knead it until it turns smooth. Make it into a small ball and let it rest in the fridge for about 30 minutes.
2. Cut the asparagus and put it in saltwater for around three minutes. Drain and put aside.
3. In another bowl, add the oil, the corn starch, silken tofu, turmeric, herbs, and black salt.
4. Mix until smooth.
5. Cut the tofu into cubes. Put some olive oil in a pan and fry the tofu for five minutes on high heat until it turns crispy.
6. Preheat the oven to 350 °F.
7. Cut the tomatoes and green onions and add the asparagus, the smoked tofu, the tomatoes, and the green onion to the mixture. Keep stirring.
8. Grease a quiche pan with butter. Put the dough into the pan and press it evenly into the bottom and the sides of the pan.
9. Add the tofu mixture, then the cherry tomatoes, and bake for about 25–30 minutes.
10. Serve warm.

20. Seitan Strips

This quick and easy recipe is enough to satiate your taste buds. Seitan is a vegetarian substitute for meat that you can use to make a variety of dishes, including Chinese, sandwiches, fries, and more.

Time: 15 minutes

Serving Size: 3–4 servings

Prep Time: 5 minutes

Cook Time: 10 minutes

Nutritional Facts/Info:

Calories	259 kcal
Carbs	11 g
Fat	11 g
Protein	29 g
Fiber	1 g

Ingredients:

- 1 pound seitan
- 2 tbsp barbecue sauce
- 2 tbsp soy sauce
- 2 tbsp balsamic vinegar
- 2-3 tbsp olive oil
- 1 to 2 tbsp water

Directions:

1. In a pan over medium-low flame, cook the seitan slices for around five minutes, until they are nicely browned from all sides.

2. Coat the seitan with soy sauce and add barbecue sauce, balsamic vinegar, and around 1–2 tablespoons of water. Coat the seitan well.

3. Cook for another two minutes, until it absorbs all the water and the seitan is completely cooked.

4. Use the meaty seitan strips to make anything you like.

Chapter 32.Non-Vegetarian Recipes for Intermittent Fasting

Indulge your taste buds with a variety of dishes. Some of these dishes are so well-liked that you'll often find foodies serving them up in the privacy of their own homes.

21.   Chicken Mascarpone

Stuffed chicken breast with mascarpone cheese and a cheese filling. Mascarpone acts as a tenderizer for the chicken and has a very subtle taste. Bake it in the oven or on the grill and serve with a white wine sauce. If desired, you may use sliced tomatoes with the mascarpone in the filling.

Time: 1 hour 15 minutes

Serving Size: 4 servings

Prep Time: 15 minutes

Cook Time: 1 hour

Nutritional Facts/Info:

Calories	197.94 kcal
Carbs	4.19 g
Fat	13.77 g
Protein	9.92 g
Fiber	0.36 g

Ingredients:

- 2 ¼ pounds chicken breast
- 1/4 cup olive oil
- 1 garlic clove
- 1 cup mascarpone cheese
- A handful of parsley
- Salt and pepper
- Ham slices (optional)

For the Sauce:

- 1/2 cup chicken stock
- 1/4 cup white wine
- 2 tbsp olive oil
- 1 lime
- Red chili flakes
- 1 tbsp butter
- Salt and pepper

Directions:

1. Mix the oil, parsley, salt, pepper, and minced garlic in a mixing bowl.

2. Coat the chicken breasts evenly to marinate.

3. Cut open the chicken breast lengthwise to form a pocket.

4. Place the ham slices and a spoonful of mascarpone inside the chicken breast, then secure the filling with a toothpick.

5. Set aside the filled chicken and repeat the process with the remaining chicken breasts.

Cooking:

1. Heat a pan and add oil and butter, wine, chicken stock, and lime juice.

2. Sprinkle salt, pepper, and chili flakes, then let it simmer while you cook the chicken.

3. Cook the chicken in a pan or on a barbecue, or you can cook the chicken in the oven at 400 degrees Fahrenheit.

4. Serve it with a spoon of prepared sauce.

22.   Chicken Quinoa and Broccoli

Creamy Chicken Quinoa and Broccoli Casserole is a healthy meal that meets your comfort food requirements. This dish is cooked from scratch, fast and simple, and packed with quality ingredients.

Time: 1 hour 15 minutes

Serving Size: 6 servings

Prep Time: 15 minutes

Cook Time: 1 hour

Nutritional Facts/Info:

Calories	317 kcal
Carbs	32.5 g
Fat	7.9 g
Protein	28.6 g
Fiber	3.5 g

Ingredients:

- 2 cups chicken broth
- 1 cup quinoa
- 1/4 cup bacon
- 1 pound boneless skinless chicken breasts
- 1/4 cup Gruyere cheese
- 3 cups broccoli florets

- 1 cup milk
- 2 cups water
- 1/2 cup flour
- 2 tsp seasoning

Directions:

1. Prepare a baking dish by greasing it liberally and preheat the oven to 400 °F. In a saucepan add the chicken broth and 1/2 cup milk and boil it on low heat. Combine the remaining 1/2 cup milk into a smooth, creamy sauce by whisking in the seasonings and flour, then pour it into the simmering liquid.

2. Stir together the first step's sauce, one cup of water, quinoa, and bacon in a casserole. Place the prepared baking dish with the batter in it. Lay the chicken pieces on top of the quinoa mixture after slicing them into thin strips. Sprinkle the seasoning over the meat. Bake for 30 minutes, uncovered.

3. While the casserole is baking, put the broccoli in boiling water for 1 minute until it becomes bright green and then run it under cold water. Place the broccoli aside.

4. Take out the casserole from the oven and check if the mixture requires more cooking. Bake it for 10–15 minutes more if needed. Once the quinoa and chicken are cooked, and the sauce has thickened substantially, add the broccoli and a little water until the mixture is creamy and smooth and easily stirred in the pan. Add the cheese and bake for 5 minutes, or until the cheese is melted, then remove from the oven.

23. Stuffed Pepper Soup

This soup, which is inspired by stuffed peppers, comes together quickly and requires just a handful of utensils. Top with anything you'd like. Cheddar cheese and tortilla chips are what we're using in this recipe, but you could use salsa, sour cream, or corn.

Time: 50 minutes

Serving Size: 4 servings

Prep Time: 25 minutes

Cook Time: 25 minutes

Nutritional Facts/Info:

Calories	570 kcal
Carbs	51 g
Fat	10 g
Protein	26 g

Fiber	6 g

Ingredients:

- 3 bell peppers
- 1 poblano pepper
- 1 pound lean ground beef
- 4 cups chicken broth
- 1 cup brown rice
- 1 tbsp extra virgin olive oil
- 1 onion and more for serving
- 2 garlic cloves
- 2 tsp cumin
- 1 tsp coriander
- 1/2 tsp pepper
- 1/4 tsp salt
- 1/4 cup fresh cilantro and more for serving
- Cheddar cheese
- Tortilla chips

Directions:

1. In a large pot, heat oil over a medium-high flame. Add the bell and poblano peppers, and onion and simmer for approximately 10 minutes until they begin to soften. Push the veggies to the side. In the center, add the meat, garlic, ground cumin, ground coriander, ground pepper, and salt and cook. Break the beef occasionally with a wooden spoon until it is no longer pink for 3–5 minutes.

2. Add the broth and rice and bring the mixture to a boil. Reduce the heat to a low simmer, cover the pot, and cook the rice for 15–20 minutes, or until it is soft. Remove from the stove and stir in the cilantro.

3. Top it with cheese, onion, cilantro, and corn chips, and serve.

24. Baked Pork Chops

Pork chops are capable of being juicy, tender, and flavorful–truly! Pork roasted in the oven will have a crispy crust and a tender inside.

Time: 30 minutes

Serving Size: 4 servings

Prep Time: 10 minutes

Cook Time: 20 minutes

Nutritional Facts/Info:

Calories	460 kcal

Carbs	1 g
Fat	33 g
Protein	39 g
Fiber	0 g

Ingredients:

- 4 pork loin chops
- Kosher salt
- 2 garlic cloves
- 1 tbsp extra virgin olive oil
- Black pepper
- 1 tbsp rosemary
- 1/2 cup butter

Directions:

1. Preheat the oven to 375 °F. Add salt and pepper seasoning to the pork chops.

2. In a small bowl, combine the butter, rosemary, and garlic with salt and pepper to taste. Set away for later.

3. Pour olive oil into an oven-safe skillet and add pork chops. Sear for 4 minutes until golden, then turn and fry for another 4 minutes. Brush heavily with garlic butter on pork chops.

25. Italian-Style Beef and Pork Meatballs

This recipe yields enough meatballs to last a few days. In addition to being a convenient supper option, they can also be used as an impromptu appetizer.

Time: 35 minutes

Serving Size: 12 servings

Prep Time: 15 minutes

Cook Time: 20 minutes

Nutritional Facts/Info:

Calories	216 kcal
Carbs	6 g
Fat	10 g
Protein	26 g
Fiber	1 g

Ingredients:

- 1 1/2 pounds ground pork
- 1 1/2 pounds ground beef
- 1/2 Parmesan cheese
- 3 eggs
- 1 cup onion
- 3/4 cup breadcrumbs
- 1 1/2 tsp salt
- 1 tsp pepper
- 1 tbsp Italian seasoning
- 3 garlic cloves
- 3/4 cup fresh parsley

Directions:

1. Preheat the oven to 450 °F and position racks in the upper and bottom thirds. Line two large rimmed baking sheets with foil and spray with cooking oil.

2. In a large bowl, mix eggs, onion, breadcrumbs, parsley, Parmesan, garlic, Italian seasoning, salt, and pepper. Add in the beef and pork. In a small bowl, mix all of the ingredients with your hands until they're well incorporated. Make 48 meatballs using a generous two teaspoons of the mixture for each. Place evenly 1 inch apart on a baking sheet.

3. Bake the meatballs for approximately 15 minutes, or until an instant-read thermometer inserted in the middle reads 165 °F.

26. Grilled Flatiron Steak with Toasted Spice Vinaigrette

Place the steaks on the top of the tomatoes. As their juices mix, the dressing will improve even more.

Time: 20 minutes

Serving Size: 4 servings

Prep Time: 5 minutes

Cook Time: 15 minutes

Nutritional Facts/Info:

Calories	540 kcal
Carbs	8 g
Fat	35 g
Protein	47 g
Fiber	3 g

Ingredients:

- 1/2 pounds skirt steak
- 4 beefsteak tomatoes
- Kosher salt

- Toasted spice vinaigrette
- 1 tbsp olive oil

Directions:

1. Make sure the grill is ready at medium heat. Rub the steak with oil and season with salt and pepper before cooking.

2. Cook each side for 4 minutes on the grill to get medium-rare steak. After cooling for 5 minutes, slice against the grain.

3. To serve, place the steak on top of the tomatoes with vinaigrette.

27. Lemon-Garlic Steak and Green Beans

In our search for a flavorful steak that is not too fatty, we usually prefer strips. The cut contains less than half the saturated fat of a ribeye, but it is softer than leaner sirloin. Cook green beans in the same pan used to sear the seasoned steak. All those delectable drippings add flavor to the beans, and there's one less pan to wash!

Time: 20 minutes

Serving Size: 4 servings

Prep Time: 0 minutes

Cook Time: 20 minutes

Nutritional Facts/Info:

Calories	215 kcal
Carbs	10 g
Fat	9 g
Protein	24 g
Fiber	3 g

Ingredients:

- 1 pound green beans
- 1 pound boneless strip steak
- 1 tbsp grapeseed or canola oil
- 1 tsp paprika
- 3 garlic cloves
- 1/2 tsp chili powder
- 1/2 tsp salt
- 2 tbsp lemon juice
- 1/2 tbsp water

Directions:

1. Add the oil, garlic, paprika, and chili powder to a small bowl and make a mixture. Apply the mixture

to the steak. Heat a big skillet to medium-high. Cook the steak, checking the temperature with an instant-read thermometer after 10 to 12 minutes, and adjust the heat if necessary to avoid smoking until the internal temperature reaches 135 °F for medium-rare. Let it lay on a clean chopping board while you prepare the next step.

2. Remove the brown pieces off the bottom of the pan with lemon juice and water. Add salt and pepper to taste for the green beans. Continue cooking for another 5 minutes, until the beans are soft, but still firm.

3. Using a sharp knife, slice the steak against the grain and serve with the green beans.

28. Egg Roll With Creamy Chili Sauce

This egg roll with a creamy chili sauce is a delicious recipe that's easy to make. In this recipe, you'll find a delicious Asian dinner that is both low carb and keto-friendly, plus a paleo slaw.

Time: 25 minutes

Serving Size: 1 serving

Prep Time: 5 minutes

Cook Time: 20 minutes

Nutritional Facts/Info:

Calories	416 kcal
Carbs	12 g
Fat	31 g
Protein	21 g
Fiber	3 g

Ingredients:

- 1 pound ground pork
- 1 14-ounce coleslaw mix
- 2 tbsp sesame oil
- 5 garlic cloves
- 6 green onions
- 1 tbsp hot sauce or sriracha
- 1 tbsp rice wine vinegar
- 1/8-1/4 tsp white or black pepper
- 3 tbsp coconut aminos or soy sauce
- 1 tsp ginger
- Salt
- Black sesame seeds

For Creamy Chili Sauce

- 1-2 tbsp hot sauce or sriracha
- 1/4 cup mayonnaise
- Salt

Directions:

1. In a big pan, heat sesame oil at a medium-high flame. Add the white sections of the green onions along with the garlic and sauté consistently for approximately 5 minutes.

2. Toss in the ground pork, hot sriracha sauce, and one tablespoon creamy chili sauce and simmer for 7 to 10 minutes until the meat turns brown and breaks up, and the sauce thickens.

3. Stir together the coleslaw mix, coconut aminos or soy sauce, rice wine vinegar, white pepper, and salt to taste. Cook for approximately 5 minutes, constantly stirring until the mixture turns soft.

4. In the meanwhile, combine 1/4 cup mayonnaise with 1-2 teaspoons of hot sauce in a small dish. Add a dash of salt to taste. In a plastic sandwich bag, add a tiny amount of creamy chili sauce to drizzle.

5. To serve, spoon a generous portion of the pork-cabbage mixture into a bowl. Slice a tiny part of the creamy chili sauce sandwich bag and pour it over the egg rolls in a bowl. Garnish with green onion pieces and black sesame seeds.

29. Vegetable Beef Soup

Tender pieces of beef, a bounty of veggies and potatoes, and a tomato broth combine to make this hearty vegetable beef soup. It's a one-pot supper that's ideal for a chilly night!

Time: 1 hour 40 minutes

Serving Size: 6 serving

Prep Time: 20 minutes

Cook Time: 1 hour 20 minutes

Nutritional Facts/Info:

Calories	367 kcal
Carbs	2 g
Fat	10 g
Protein	40 g
Fiber	4 g

Ingredients:

- 2 pounds beef stew meat
- 7 cups beef broth
- 28 oz diced tomatoes
- 2 tsp garlic
- 1/2 cup onion
- 3 carrots
- 2 stalks celery
- 2 cups russet potato
- 1/2 cup frozen peas
- 1/2 cup frozen corn
- 3/4 cup frozen green beans
- 1 bay leaf
- 1 tbsp olive oil
- 1 1/2 tsp Italian seasoning
- 2 tbsp parsley
- Salt and pepper

Directions:

1. In a large skillet, heat the olive oil to a medium-high temperature. Add salt and pepper according to taste to season the stew meat.

2. Place half of the meat in a single layer in the pan. Fry for 3–4 minutes on each side, or until it turns brown. Repeat the step with the remaining meat. Keep the steak warm by placing it on a platter and covering it.

3. Pan-fry the onion, carrot, and celery. Cook for around 4 to 5 minutes until it turns soft. Cook it for 30 seconds after adding the garlic.

4. Add the meat back to the skillet, and combine the tomatoes, Italian spice, bay leaf, and beef stock, and cook until the meat is no longer pink. Put on low heat and simmer for a few minutes with the mixture.

5. Cook the meat for 60 minutes or until it is tender.

6. Now add in your potatoes. Make sure you cut them into big chunks before cooking.

7. Continue cooking for another 20 minutes or more until the potatoes are fork-tender.

8. Add corn, peas, and green beans at this time and cook for 5 minutes. Season with salt and pepper.

9. Discard the bay leaf. Sprinkle with fresh parsley before serving.

30. Apple, Pork, and Miso Noodle Soup

This simple noodle soup is flavored with apples and mild white miso. Adding a splash of the spicy sauce gives it an extra kick without overpowering the dish's taste. Include a watercress salad on the side.

Time: 35 minutes

Serving Size: 4 servings

Prep Time:

Cook Time:

Nutritional Facts/Info:

Calories	406 kcal
Carbs	57.3 g
Fat	8.9 g
Protein	26.9 g
Fiber	8.3 g

Ingredients:

- ½ cup white miso
- 8 oz whole wheat noodles
- 2 cups chicken broth
- 12 oz lean ground pork
- 1 tbsp canola oil
- 2 apples
- 4 cups water

Directions:

1. Heat oil in a saucepan and add in the pork, and cook until the meat is no longer pink, approximately for two minutes. Toss in apples, stir and cook for an additional 2 minutes.

2. In a separate pan, boil the water and broth to cook the noodles, adding salt and pepper to taste.

3. When the noodles are almost done, gather up roughly half of the cooking liquid from the pan and blend with miso. Remove the pan from the heat and add the miso mixture. Now serve the soup.

31. Honey Mustard Salmon

This recipe for healthy baked Honey Mustard Salmon is quick, flavorful, and very simple to prepare. The honey mustard glaze on top of this dish is what elevates it to culinary greatness. Honey and mustard are the obvious ingredients in the glaze, but there are also a few more that give it a unique flavor. Salad, rice, or steamed vegetables are all good side dishes to add for a proper supper.

Time: 30 minutes

Serving Size: 4 servings

Prep Time: 10 minutes

Cook Time: 20 minutes

Nutritional Facts/Info:

Calories	415 kcal

Carbs	8 g
Fat	22 g
Protein	45 g
Fiber	1 g

Ingredients:

- 2 pounds boneless salmon
- 1 1/2 tbsp mustard
- 1 1/2 tbsp honey
- 2 tbsp olive oil
- 1 tbsp lemon juice
- 2 garlic cloves
- Handful fresh parsley
- Salt and pepper

Directions:

1. Add mustard, honey, garlic, olive oil, and lemon juice into a small bowl and whisk well with salt and pepper.

2. Using aluminum foil, line a large baking sheet. Place the salmon filet in the center of the foil-lined baking sheet.

3. Apply the honey mustard mixture to the fish using a basting brush. Allow 30 minutes for the marinade to work.

4. Preheat the oven to 375 °F while the salmon gets marinated.

5. Bake for 20–25 minutes and check if the salmon flakes easily with a fork. Take it out when it does.

6. Garnish with parsley and serve.

32. Beef Stir-Fry With Baby Bok Choy

A single wok can cook everything for this quick and nutritious beef stir-fry, making meal prep and cleanup a breeze! Go to your local grocery store and look for oyster sauce. You'll love how it enhances the taste of this recipe.

Time: 25 minutes

Serving Size: 4 servings

Prep Time: 0 minutes

Cook Time: 25 minutes

Nutritional Facts/Info:

Calories	247 kcal
Carbs	6.3 g

Fat	12.8 g
Protein	25.5 g
Fiber	1.1 g

Ingredients:

- 12 oz beef flank steak
- 1 pound baby bok choy
- 3 tbsp unsalted chicken broth
- 1 tbsp ginger
- 1 1/2 tsp reduced-sodium soy sauce
- 1 tbsp vegetable oil
- 1 tsp sesame oil
- 1 tsp cornstarch
- 1 tsp dry sherry
- 2 tbsp oyster sauce

Directions:

1. Slice the beef with grain into 2-inch-wide strips. Cut each strip into 1/4-inch-thick slices by cutting it against the grain. In a medium bowl, combine the beef, ginger, soy sauce, sherry, and cornstarch. Mix until the cornstarch is no longer visible. Lightly coat the beef with sesame oil while stirring.

2. Use a small bowl for mixing the oyster sauce and sherry. And a pinch of salt and pepper and set aside.

3. Make sure your carbon-steel wok or stainless-steel pan is hot enough to evaporate a drop of water in less than a second. Pour in some vegetable oil and swirl it around. Add the beef in an even layer and cook for approximately 1 minute until brown. Use a metal spatula to stir-fry lightly, but don't overcook it. Now, transfer it to a plate.

4. Add the bok choy and broth and cook it covered for 1–2 minutes, or until bright green and almost all the liquid is absorbed. The bok choy should still be crisp-tender, so return the beef to the pan and stir-fry for almost 1 minute with the reserved sauce.

33. Ground Beef Chili

This dish is simple to prepare, nutritious, and spicy. A portion of ideal comfort food on a chilly day is flavorful and has protein content. This recipe for Ground Beef Chili, made with beef, kidney beans, tomatoes, garlic, and a slew of spices, is packed with flavor. With this one-pot recipe, you can have dinner on the table in less than 30 minutes.

Time: 35 minutes

Serving Size: 6 servings

Prep Time: 5 minutes

Cook Time: 30 minutes

Nutritional Facts/Info:

Calories	286 kcal
Carbs	31 g
Fat	8 g
Protein	26 g
Fiber	10 g

Ingredients:

- 1 14 oz can crushed tomatoes
- 1 15 oz can diced tomatoes
- 1/4 cup tomato paste
- 1 15 oz can kidney beans
- 2 cups beef broth
- 1 pound ground beef
- 3 tbsp chili powder
- 1 1/2 tsp ground cumin
- 1/2 tsp oregano
- 1 tbsp olive oil
- 1 yellow onion
- 4 garlic clove

For Toppings:

- Cheddar cheese
- Cilantro
- Sour cream

Directions:

1. Heat the oil in a saucepan, add the onion and cook it for about 4 minutes, or until it becomes translucent. Add the garlic and continue to cook for another one minute.

2. Toss in the ground beef and simmer for approximately 5 minutes, stirring regularly to break it up and until brown.

3. Mix in all of the seasonings (chili powder, cumin, and oregano).

4. Stir in the broth, kidney beans, crushed tomatoes, diced tomatoes, and tomato paste.

5. Simmer for approximately 20 minutes over medium heat, stirring occasionally.

6. Season with salt and pepper to taste. Garnish with optional toppings if desired before serving.

34. Turkey Meatloaf

This lean ground turkey meatloaf dish is flavorful, delicious, and simple to make.

Time: 1 hour

Serving Size: 1/4 serving

Prep Time: 5 minutes

Cook Time: 55 minutes

Nutritional Facts/Info:

Calories	259 kcal
Carbs	14 g
Fat	5 g
Protein	37 g
Fiber	1.5 g

Ingredients:

- 1 1/2 lb ground turkey
- 1/2 cup gluten-free breadcrumbs
- 1 egg
- 1 tsp marjoram
- 1 tsp kosher salt
- 1 tsp olive oil
- 1/2 onion
- 2 tsp Worcestershire sauce
- 1/4 cup plus 2 tbsp ketchup

Directions:

1. Preheat the oven at 350 °F.
2. Mix 2 tablespoons of ketchup with 2 tablespoons of Worcestershire sauce in a small bowl.
3. Heat olive oil and onion in a small pan over low heat until translucent for about 3 to 5 minutes, then remove from heat.
4. Add turkey, onion, breadcrumbs, egg, and 1/4 cup ketchup to a medium bowl along with salt and marjoram.
5. Fill a loaf pan or shape it into a loaf and bake on a baking pan with the ingredients. Add a spoonful of sauce to the dish.
6. Bake, uncovered, for 55–60 minutes, then remove from oven and cool for 5 minutes before slicing.

35. Skillet Ravioli Lasagna

You don't need to layer or mix anything for this simple inside-out ravioli lasagna. It's comfort food for your busy weeknights. You may use ground turkey in place of the beef in this recipe. Make sure to look for fresh mozzarella balls in your local supermarket's specialty cheese area.

Time: 20 minutes

Serving Size: 6 serving

Prep Time: 0 minutes

Cook Time: 20 minutes

Nutritional Facts/Info:

Calories	483 kcal
Carbs	33.5 g
Fat	20.1 g
Protein	38 g
Fiber	3.1 g

Ingredients:

- 1 pound lean ground beef
- 1 24 oz package frozen cheese ravioli
- 1 28 oz can no-salt crushed tomatoes
- 8 oz mozzarella balls
- 1/4 tsp basil
- 1/4 tsp ground pepper
- 1 1/2 tsp oregano
- 1/2 tsp garlic powder
- 1/2 tsp salt

Directions:

1. Preheat the broiler, then boil a large pot of water. Cook the ravioli according to the package instructions, drain, and put aside.
2. Over medium-high heat, sauté ground beef until it is cooked thoroughly for 4 to 5 minutes. Crumble the meat with the back of a wooden spoon as it cooks. Season it with oregano, garlic powder, and pepper.
3. Add tomatoes, and basil, and boil it. Fold in half of the mozzarella balls and the cooked ravioli.
4. Top with the rest of the mozzarella balls over the pasta. Carefully place the pan in the oven. Bake for 2–3 minutes, until the cheese melts.

Chapter 33.Snack Recipes for Intermittent Fasting

If you're feeling a bit hungry and are looking for something to snack on, try one of these tasty, healthy snacks to satisfy your hunger. You can easily make all of these nutrient-rich snacks at home, which can save you both time and money.

36. Mango Salsa

Fresh mango salsa is ready in less than 30 minutes, tastes fantastic, and is a cinch to prepare. Sweet and spicy flavors are perfectly balanced in this dish to enthrall your taste buds. Instead of tomatoes, as in traditional salsa, this savory salsa uses sweet, juicy mangoes. The jalapeno adds just the right amount of kick without overpowering the other flavors. The ingredients used in this dish make it an appealing appetizer you can have at any time.

Time: 25 minutes

Serving Size: 4 servings

Prep Time: 25 minutes

Cook Time: 0 minutes

Nutritional Facts/Info:

Calories	221 kcal
Carbs	55 g
Fat	1 g
Protein	3 g
Fiber	6 g

Ingredients:

- 3 ripe mangos, diced
- 1/2 cup red bell pepper
- 1 jalapeño pepper, without seeds
- 1/4 cup red onion
- 2 tbsp fresh lime juice
- 1/3 tsp chili powder
- 1/4 cup fresh cilantro
- 1/4 tsp salt, or to taste

Directions:

1. Cut the mango and bell pepper into small pieces.
2. Finely dice the jalapeño and onion. Chop the cilantro as well.
3. In a big bowl, add all of the ingredients together. Drizzle some lime juice and salt.
4. Gently mix everything with a large spoon or rubber spatula.
5. Let it chill in the refrigerator for 15–30 minutes before serving to let it absorb all the flavor.

37. Cinnamon Popcorn

Mood-lifting, immune-boosting, and antioxidant-rich foods abound in this cinnamon popcorn snack mix. It's the ideal back-to-school treat for students of all ages. All the ingredients picked for this recipe are full of nutrients and so filling that you won't be thinking about food before dinner. The best part? No cooking needed!

Time: 5 minutes

Serving Size: 7 servings

Prep Time: 5 minutes

Cook Time: 0 minutes

Nutritional Facts/Info:

Calories	598 kcal
Carbs	18 g
Fat	10 g
Protein	12 g
Fiber	8 g

Ingredients:

- 5 cups popped popcorn
- 3/4 cup pepitas
- 3/4 cup sunflower seeds
- 1/4 cup dried cranberries tart cherries
- 1/4 cup dried blueberries

Directions:

1. In a bowl, mix the popcorn, sunflower seeds/walnuts, pepitas, dried cranberries, and blueberries.
2. Enjoy right away.
3. To use it for a longer period, put it in airtight containers.

38. Vada Pav

Vada Pav hails from the West Indian state of Maharashtra and is a popular national dish. In the 1960s and 1970s, it was a staple food for the industrial workers in Mumbai's central neighborhood. It is an affordable, tasty, and easy-to-prepare snack that your taste buds will love for sure!

Time: 60 minutes

Serving Size: 6 servings

Prep Time: 15 minutes

Cook Time: 45 minutes

Nutritional Facts/Info:

Calories	706 kcal
Carbs	117 g
Fat	20 g
Protein	19 g
Fiber	13 g

Ingredients:

- 10 medium potatoes
- 3 pepper chilis
- 2 tsp garlic paste
- 1 tsp ginger paste
- 1/2 tsp turmeric
- 6 to 7 curry leaves
- 1/2 tsp black mustard seeds
- 1/4 tsp salt, or to taste
- 2 cups gram flour
- 1 cup tamarind chutney
- 1 cup green chutney
- 1/3 cup oil
- 6 pav buns, or burger buns
- 1/2 cup garlic chutney

Directions:

1. In a bowl, add the gram flour with water and salt and mix it to make a thick paste without any lumps. To avoid making the batter runny, add water slowly and stop once you get a thick, soupy consistency. Set it aside.

2. Add the garlic and ginger pastes and the green chilies to the food processor and make a smooth paste.

3. Boil the potatoes and let them cool. Once they are done, mash them with a fork.

4. Mix the paste with the boiled and mashed potatoes. Add salt for seasoning.

5. In a pan, add two tablespoons of oil on medium heat. Add the curry leaves, mustard seeds, and turmeric powder.

6. Once the seeds stop spluttering, add to the potato mixture and mix.

7. Divide the mixture into medium balls. Press them slightly with your hands.

8. Put oil for frying on medium heat.

9. Once it is hot, dip the potato balls one by one into the batter made earlier and coat well. Deep fry the coated balls until golden. Drain the excess oil.

10. Take a pav bun and cut it in half, leaving one end joined. Add in the chutneys. Put a potato ball on each bun and fold it over.

11. Serve hot.

39. Potato Salad

This classic potato salad is flavorful, appetizing, and a party favorite. Serve it at your next summer get together, and be ready for tons of compliments! You can use vegan mayo instead of regular mayo without compromising on the taste. Add celery and onion for that extra crunch and olives (or pickles) for a salty kick!

Time: 30 minutes

Serving Size: 8 servings

Prep Time: 15 minutes

Cook Time: 15 minutes

Nutritional Facts/Info:

Calories	147 kcal
Carbs	32 g
Fat	0 g
Protein	4 g
Fiber	4 g

Ingredients:

- 5–6 potatoes
- 1 (6 oz) can of black olives
- 1/2 cup onion
- 3/4 cup celery
- 1 1/2 cups mayo
- 1/2 tsp salt
- 1/3 tsp paprika
- 1/4 tsp celery seed

- Salt and pepper

Directions:

1. Wash the potatoes to remove any dirt. Cut them without removing the skins, leaving smaller potatoes as they are.

2. Add them to a big pot and add water just enough to cover them. Let it come to a boil and add 1–2 teaspoons of salt. Cook for about 8–10 minutes or until they are tender. Drain the water and set aside.

3. Once they are cooled, remove the skins.

4. Chop the potatoes into small pieces and add them to a bowl.

5. Add salt and toss it to mix.

6. Add the other ingredients and mix to combine everything well.

7. Put more salt and pepper if required. Let it sit for an hour.

8. Before serving, top it with some paprika for extra flavor.

9. Enjoy!

40. Baba Ganoush

This simple Baba Ganoush is a wonderful dip or appetizer that is both nutritious and delicious. It goes well with pita, naan bread, or falafel and tabbouleh as a dipping sauce. And it doesn't get any easier than this! It takes about 50 minutes to prepare in total. When it comes to baking, however, the recipe requires a total of 40 minutes, during which you don't need to do anything.

Time: 50 minutes

Serving Size: 6 servings

Prep Time: 10 minutes

Cook Time: 40 minutes

Nutritional Facts/Info:

Calories	162 kcal
Carbs	12 g
Fat	12 g
Protein	3 g
Fiber	5 g

Ingredients:

- 2 medium eggplants
- 2 cloves of garlic
- 3 tbsp lemon juice

- 3 tbsp extra virgin olive oil
- 1/4 cup tahini
- 3/4 tsp salt
- 2 tbsp parsley

Directions:

1. Preheat the oven to 350 degrees Fahrenheit.

2. Cut the eggplant in half. Put parchment paper over the baking tray and put the eggplants with the flesh side facing up.

3. Brush with some olive oil.

4. Bake for around 40 minutes. In the last 10–15 minutes, cover the eggplants minutes to avoid overcooking.

5. Let them cool. Meanwhile, add the other ingredients to a food processor.

6. Take out the flesh of the eggplant and add it to the mixture.

7. Add chopped parsley, red pepper flakes, and olive oil.

8. Serve with pita bread.

41. Garlic Herb Tomatoes

Cherry tomatoes blend with garlic and herbs in this simple and irresistibly delicious recipe. They are so versatile that you can use them as a topping for any dish.

Time: 20 minutes

Serving Size: 2 servings

Prep Time: 10 minutes

Cook Time: 10 minutes

Nutritional Facts/Info:

Calories	421 kcal
Carbs	25 g
Fat	31 g
Protein	7 g
Fiber	8 g

Ingredients:

- 2 tbsp olive oil
- 1 tsp dried basil
- 4 cups cherry tomatoes
- ½ tsp dried parsley
- 1 tsp dried oregano

- ¼ tsp red pepper flakes
- Salt, to taste
- 3 cloves garlic, minced

Directions:

1. Put a large pan over a medium heat and add some olive oil.
2. Add the basil, parsley, oregano, and red pepper flakes and sauté until it turns fragrant for around 30 seconds.
3. Add the tomatoes and sea salt. Put the flame to medium-high, and cook for around 6–10 minutes or until the tomatoes get a light golden brown color. Stir them a bit to prevent them from sticking to the pan.
4. Add the garlic and cook for one more minute until the garlic turns soft.
5. Let it cool.
6. Serve with pasta, salad, hummus, etc.

42. Roasted Chickpeas

Snacking on roasted chickpeas is both delicious and beneficial to your health. Their mild spiciness and extremely easy preparation make them the perfect on-the-go snack. They're ideal for a variety of occasions, including parties, watching TV, long drives, and more.

Time: 40 minutes

Serving Size: 4 servings

Prep Time: 5 minutes

Cook Time: 35 minutes

Nutritional Facts/Info:

Calories	263 kcal
Carbs	31 g
Fat	11 g
Protein	11 g
Fiber	10 g

Ingredients:

- 2 cans chickpeas, drained
- 1 tsp smoked paprika powder
- 2 tbsp olive oil
- 1/2 tsp salt
- 1 tsp garlic powder

Directions:

1. Preheat the oven to 450 degrees Fahrenheit.
2. Dry the chickpeas by wiping them with a paper towel. Stir together chickpeas, olive oil, salt, paprika powder, and salt in a bowl. Increase or decrease the quantity as per your liking.
3. Bake for 30–40 minutes, stirring occasionally, until the chickpeas are golden and crunchy. Make sure to not overheat.
4. Enjoy hot or let them cool before serving.

43. Nacho Potato Wedges

These nacho-loaded potato wedges are a crowd pleaser, no matter the occasion. Vegan yummy cheese, cherry tomato, taco crumbles, avocado, scallions, jalapenos, and vegan sour cream are all layered on top of baked and seasoned potato wedges. What could be better than this?

Time: 30 minutes

Serving Size: 6 servings

Prep Time: 10 minutes

Cook Time: 20 minutes

Nutritional Facts/Info:

Calories	356 kcal
Carbs	35 g
Fat	18 g
Protein	10 g
Fiber	13 g

Ingredients:

- 6 large potatoes
- 2 to 3 tbsp oil
- ¼ small onion
- ¼ cup cilantro
- ¾ cup walnuts*
- 1 tsp apple cider vinegar
- 2 ½ tbsp taco seasoning
- 1 pint cherry tomatoes
- 1 tbsp taco seasoning
- Sea salt, to taste

Directions:

For the potato wedges:

1. Preheat the oven to 400 degrees Fahrenheit. Line two baking trays with parchment paper.

2. Slice the potatoes into wedges. Divide them evenly between parchment-lined pans, drizzle some oil, add some taco seasoning, and toss to mix well.

3. Spread evenly on the pan, leaving a little space between each wedge.

4. Bake for about 40–45 minutes, flipping in between, or until they turn tender and golden.

For the Cherry Tomato Pico de Gallo

5. In a bowl, mix the onion, tomatoes, and cilantro. Add some sea salt for seasoning.

6. Keep in the fridge.

For the Walnut Taco Crumbles

7. Add walnuts, taco seasoning, and vinegar to a food processor. Pulse a few times and process for 30 seconds or until it has a crumbly texture.

8. Heat a skillet on medium-high heat. Add the crumbles and toast for about 3–4 minutes, or until they are golden, stirring in between.

9. Let it cool before serving.

44. Breakfast Burritos

These oil-free and quick vegan breakfast burritos feature a Mexican flair and a ton of flavor. And by easy, I mean uncomplicated. Since when does one need a million steps before they can have breakfast? All you need are a few simple ingredients and 30 minutes of your time to whip these up.

Time: 50 minutes

Serving Size: 5 servings

Prep Time: 10 minutes

Cook Time: 40 minutes

Nutritional Facts/Info:

Calories	356 kcal
Carbs	35 g
Fat	18 g
Protein	10 g
Fiber	13 g

Ingredients:

- 1 cup cooked chickpeas
- 2 cups potatoes, sliced
- 2 cups bell peppers
- 1 cup corn
- 1/8-1/4 tsp ground chipotle spice
- 1 cup salsa
- 1 tsp ground cumin
- 1/2 tsp salt

For avocado cumin cream:

- 1 large avocado
- 1/2 tsp ground cumin
- 2 tbsp salsa
- 1/2 tbsp lime juice
- 1/4 tsp fine sea salt
- Large tortillas
- Fresh jalapenos, optional

Directions:

1. Preheat the oven to 400 degrees Fahrenheit. Line a baking sheet with parchment paper.

2. Spread the potatoes evenly and season with salt and pepper. Make sure you cut your potatoes to about 1/4 inch. Bake for 20 minutes until they turn brown.

3. Chop the bell peppers into 2-inch strips. Start cooking the bell peppers in the last 10 minutes of the potatoes.

4. In a pan, add 1/4 cup water and add the bell peppers. Over medium heat, cook for around 5–8 minutes until all the water has evaporated.

5. Add the salsa, chickpeas, corn, cumin, and chipotle pepper. Cook for 5–10 minutes until the sauce has thickened. Add the potatoes last and remove them from the heat.

6. For the avocado cumin cream, add all the ingredients in a food processor or hand blender. Blend until smooth.

7. Add the veggie mixture to the tortillas with the avocado cream on top.

8. Enjoy!

Chapter 34.Dessert Recipes for Intermittent Fasting

Who doesn't crave something sweet at times? But the sugar levels in all those desserts stops us from having them. Even if we have them once in a while, we go on a guilt trip that is hard to come back from. Intermittent fasting allows you to satisfy your cravings without guilt. Try out these six insanely delicious and sugar-free desserts that you can make with the ingredients available at hand.

45. Peanut Butter Oatmeal Bars

These Peanut Butter Oatmeal Bars are a delight for any person. The irresistible chewy texture, a lovely peanutty flavor, and a downpour of chocolate on top are what everyone craves. These no-bake bars will bring a blissful and healthier dessert option to your menu.

Time: 15 minutes

Serving Size: 20 bars (4 x 5 inches)

Prep Time: 15 minutes

Cook Time: 0 minutes

Nutritional Facts/Info:

Calories (per serving)	171 kcal
Carbs	21.4 g
Fat	7.2 g
Protein	5 g
Fiber	2.4 g

Ingredients:

- 1 cup creamy peanut butter (no sugar added) or sunflower butter (for nut-free)
- 4 cup old fashioned rolled oats
- ½ cup honey or ½ cup agave syrup (for vegan)
- ½ teaspoon cinnamon
- 1 to 2 ounces dark chocolate (1/8 to 1/4 cup chocolate chips)
- ½ teaspoon kosher salt

Directions:

1. Start by mixing peanut butter, oats, cinnamon, honey, and salt in a bowl. If you feel the mixture is dry and does not become sticky, try adding more peanut butter and/or honey. Note that peanut butter from different brands works differently.
2. The next step involves adding a sheet of parchment paper to a 9 x 9 pan. Pour the mixture into the pan and firmly press it to make an even layer. You can do so by rolling a small glass over the top.
3. Finally, freeze the bars for about 10 minutes. Take the pan out of the freezer and lift the bars using the parchment paper. You can cut them into 40 small or 20 regular rectangles (4 x 5 rows).
4. The final step is to melt the chocolate using a microwave. When using the microwave, give the chocolate short bursts of 10 seconds and stir after each. Do not overheat the chocolate, as overheating can seize it up. Finally, drizzle the melted chocolate over the oatmeal bars and let them cool.
5. You can consume the bars right away or refrigerate them for about 1 hour to get a more solid texture.

46. Chocolate Covered Banana Bites

The concept of Chocolate Covered Bananas is not new or revolutionary. But, its taste and crispy nature make it an ideal healthy dessert option. This ultra-delicious dish brings out the sweetness of dark chocolate and the magic of icy banana pieces.

Time: 1 hour 30 minutes

Serving Size: 30 to 35 bites

Prep Time: 1 hour 30 minutes

Cook Time: 0 minutes

Nutritional Facts/Info:

Calories (per bite)	48 kcal
Carbs	6.6 g
Fat	2.6 g
Protein	0.6 g
Fiber	0.7 g

Ingredients:

- 1 ½ cup dark chocolate chips (roughly 5 ounces)
- 1 pinch of salt
- 2 ripe medium-sized bananas
- 1 tbsp refined coconut oil
- 2 tbsp each of crushed pistachios, crushed peanuts, and sprinkles (optional)

Directions:

1. Start by cutting the bananas into 1/4-inch rounds. Place them over a baking sheet and give a 45-minute freeze to the pieces.

2. Take a pot of parboiling water. Now, place chocolate, salt, and coconut oil in a glass and put it into the simmering pot to melt the chocolate. Cautiously stir the mix while also ensuring that water does not mix with chocolate. You can also use a microwave to achieve the same.

3. Using a fork, dip each frozen banana slice into the jar and remove the excess chocolate. After this, transfer each piece to the baking sheet using your fingers. If toppings are used, immediately add them because chocolate freezes quickly. Having more chocolate would make the dipping process much easier for you.

4. Transfer the newly-made chocolate covered bananas into a freezer and give them a 30-minute freeze.

47. Sauteed Apples

Want a dessert that takes just a fraction of your time to prepare? If yes, then there's no other better option than sautéed apples! Neither baking nor advanced preparation is required for this delicious dessert. Just get some apple slices, sauté them well in spices and butter, and you are ready with the dish. Adding vanilla ice cream as a topping would bring the best out of this dessert.

Time: 10 minutes

Serving Size: 4 servings

Prep Time: 5 minutes

Cook Time: 5 minutes

Nutritional Facts/Info:

Calories (per serving)	188 kcal
Carbs	29.6 g
Fat	8.9 g
Protein	0.5 g
Fiber	4 g

Ingredients:

- 3 firm large tart-sweet apples
- ½ tsp ginger
- 1 ½ tbsp brown sugar
- 1 ½ tsp cinnamon
- 1/2 tbsp granulated sugar

- 3 tbsp butter (or coconut oil for vegan)
- ¼ tsp nutmeg
- Vanilla ice cream or vegan cinnamon ice cream
- ½ tbsp Cointreau (optional)

Directions:

1. Start by slicing the apples into ¼-inch pieces. You need not peel the fruit unless you want to. Take a bowl and stir the sliced apples with cinnamon, brown and granulated sugars, nutmeg, and ginger.

2. Take a pan and medium heat the butter until it turns brown (about 2 minutes). Finally, add the apples and constantly sauté the mix for 4-5 minutes until you get a crispy result. If using Cointreau, add it now and further cook for 20 seconds. Serve the sautéed apples with vanilla ice cream.

48. Healthy Cookies

What else would be better than the good ol' cookies? Furthermore, if the cookies are healthy, no one stops you from binge eating them. The recipe below contains all health-beneficial ingredients which taste like a treat. In fact, these cookies are refined sugar-free and butter-free, making them a healthy dessert choice for both kids and adults.

Time: 30 minutes

Serving Size: 20 cookies

Prep Time: 15 minutes

Cook Time: 15 minutes

Nutritional Facts/Info:

Calories	120 kcal
Carbs	16.5 g
Fat	4.9 g
Protein	3.2 g
Fiber	1.9 g

Ingredients:

- 2 cups old fashioned oats
- ¼ cup shredded unsweetened coconut
- ½ cup cashew butter (or sunflower butter)
- 1 cup Medjool dates
- 1 egg
- 2 teaspoons vanilla
- ½ teaspoon baking soda
- ¼ cup plain or Greek yogurt
- ¼ teaspoon kosher salt

- ¼ cup mini chocolate chips
- 1 teaspoon cinnamon

Directions:

1. Before pouring the ingredients, you will need to preheat the oven to 350 degrees Fahrenheit. Place coconut in a dry skillet and medium heat it. Shake, stir, and heat the pan until the coconut turns golden brown (about 3 minutes). Once completed, transfer the coconut onto a plate. Stay near the stove as they can burn quickly.

2. Transform the old fashioned oats into a flour using a food processor. Then, remove the oats and add nut butter, salt, Medjool dates (after removing the pits), and vanilla. Process until you get a combined and crumbly mixture.

3. Add egg and yogurt to the mix and pulse it.

4. Similarly, pulse the oat flour, baking soda, cinnamon, and remaining whole oats until you form a thick dough. Mix the toasted coconut and chocolate chips in as well.

5. Finally, make 20 small balls and place them on a parchment-lined cookie sheet. Gently pour the remaining 1 tbsp of chocolate chips onto the cookies.

6. Finally, bake the cookies until golden brown for about 12–15 minutes. Rotate after every 7 minutes and allow them to cool after the time passes.

7. Enjoy!

49. Chocolate Pudding

Like sautéed apples, you need to apply minimal effort to make these healthy chocolate puddings. Just by investing a few minutes of your time, you will create something unimaginably tasty. The sweetness of cocoa and Greek yogurt will leave you craving more.

Time: 2 minutes

Serving Size: 1 serving

Prep Time: 2 minutes

Cook Time: 0 minutes

Nutritional Facts/Info:

Calories	198 kcal
Carbs	30.3 g
Fat	6.4 g
Protein	10.9 g
Fiber	3.2 g

Ingredients:

- ½ cup Greek yogurt
- 1 ½ tbsp maple syrup
- 2 tbsp dark cocoa powder

Directions:

1. Pour all the ingredients into a bowl and mix them well. At first, you will notice a thick texture, but the cocoa powder will become smoother as you mix. If you feel that the yogurt is thick, add ½ to 1 tbsp water to get a lighter texture. (Add more maple or cocoa powder to taste.)

2. Your healthy and delicious chocolate pudding is done!

50. Lemon Cookie Tarts

This no-bake lemon tart made with delicious berries and fruits is a perfect summer treat! Make your own and enjoy it while chilling by the poolside.

Time: 2 hours 30 minutes

Serving Size: 1 serving

Prep Time: 2 minutes

Cook Time: 0 minutes

Nutritional Facts/Info:

Calories	375 kcal
Carbs	27 g
Fat	27 g
Protein	14.5 g
Fiber	4.6 g

Ingredients:

For the crust:

- 2 cups walnuts
- 7–12 whole Medjool dates
- 1/4 tsp salt

For the filling:

- 12 ounces tofu
- 1/2 tsp vanilla extract
- 1/4 cup maple syrup (or honey or nectar)
- Juice of one lemon
- 1 1/2 cups mixed berries

Directions:

1. Press tofu while you prepare your crust.

2. Pulse your walnuts for a minute or two in the processor.

3. Put in your soaked dates and pulse it with the walnuts for another minute.

4. Line 4 3/4-inch tart pans with parchment paper. Add the crust mixture to the tarts one by one and press firmly to spread throughout.

5. Add drained tofu, vanilla, lemon juice, and sweetener of your choice and blend until you get a creamy texture, scraping down the edges. Add or reduce ingredients to increase the level of tartness.

6. Remove crust from the fridge and add the lemon filling. Chill to set. When serving, top with fruit and enjoy!

21-Day Meal Plan for Intermittent Fasting

Now that we have looked over the recipes, let's dive into the 21-day meal plan for intermittent fasting. This easy-to-follow plan combines the meals that are mentioned above, including snacks and desserts. You can also tweak it according to your preference, but make sure to keep the calorie count in mind.

If you follow the plan rigorously, you are sure to shed weight and, more importantly, feel healthier and happier with your body.

Days	Meal 1	Meal 2	Meal 3	Dessert/Snacks
Day 1	Mexican Quinoa	Vegetarian Casserole	Vegan Tofu Barbeque	Mango Salsa
Day 2	Oats Veggie Tots	Asian Fusion Tacos	Chicken Mascarpone	Chocolate Covered Banana Bites
Day 3	Egg Roll With Creamy Chili Sauce	Lentil Meatballs	Acapulco Slaw	Roasted Chickpeas
Day 4	Vegan Fettuccine Alfredo	Vegetarian Pad Thai	Pasta Salad	Cinnamon Popcorn
Day 5	Italian-Style Beef and Pork Meatballs	Baked Pork Chops	Stuffed Pepper Soup	Garlic Herb Tomatoes
Day 6	Vegetarian Shepherd's Pie	Grilled Flatiron Steak with Toasted Spice Vinaigrette	Honey Mustard Salmon	Sauteed Apples
Day 7	Vegan Quiche	White Bean Salad	Skillet Ravioli Lasagna	Vada Pav
Day 8	Beef Stir-Fry With Baby Bok Choy	Avocado Roast with Balsamic Drizzle	Vegan Summer Rolls	Peanut Butter Oatmeal Bars
Day 9	Skillet Ravioli Lasagna	Apple, Pork, and Miso Noodle Soup	Pasta Salad	Potato Salad
Day 10	Tofu and Spinach Scramble	Seitan Strips with the soup of your choice	Black Beans with Lime Rice	Baba Ganoush
Day 11	Grilled Flatiron Steak with Toasted Spice Vinaigrette	Vegetarian Pad Thai	Lentil Soup	Nacho Potato Wedges
Day 12	Avocado Roast with Balsamic Drizzle	Turkey Meatloaf	Vegan Thai Curry	Breakfast Burritos
Day 13	Vegan Quiche	Skillet Ravioli Lasagna	Ground Beef Chili	Lemon Cookie Tarts

Day 14	Vegan Summer Rolls	Honey Mustard Salmon	Italian-Style Beef and Pork Meatballs	Cinnamon Popcorn
Day 15	Asian Fusion Tacos	White Bean Salad	Apple, Pork, and Miso Noodle Soup	Healthy Cookies
Day 16	Acapulco Slaw	Chicken Mascarpone	Black Beans with Lime Rice	Peanut Butter Oatmeal Bars
Day 17	Vada Pav	Lemon-Garlic Steak and Green Beans	Vegan Tofu Barbeque	Chocolate Pudding
Day 18	Tofu and Spinach Scramble	Vegan Thai Curry	Egg Roll With Creamy Chili Sauce	Mango Salsa
Day 19	Oats Veggie Tots	Baked Pork Chops	Vegan Fettuccine Alfredo	Sauteed Apples
Day 20	Vegetarian Shepherd's Pie	Ground Beef Chili	Vegan Tofu Barbeque	Chocolate Pudding
Day 21	Mexican Quinoa	Vegan Quiche	Skillet Ravioli Lasagna	Baba Ganoush

References

Bond Brill, J. (2021, March 24). *10 Superfoods to include when intermittent fasting.* Dummies. https://www.dummies.com/article/body-mind-spirit/physical-health-well-being/diet-nutrition/intermittent-fasting/10-superfoods-to-include-when-intermittent-fasting-275834/

Intermittent fasting food list: What to eat and avoid. (2019, September 19). DoFasting. https://dofasting.com/blog/intermittent-fasting-food-list/

Kubala, J. (2021, April 23). *9 potential intermittent fasting side effects.* Healthline. https://www.healthline.com/nutrition/intermittent-fasting-side-effects

Tarnopolsky, M. A. (2008). Sex Differences in Exercise Metabolism and the Role of 17-Beta Estradiol. *Medicine & science in sports & exercise, 40*(4), 648–654. https://doi.org/10.1249/mss.0b013e31816212ff

Thierry. (2020, April 7). *Intermittent fasting vs. 8 other diets: The complete comparison.* Intermittent Dieter. https://intermittentdieter.com/intermittent-fasting-vs-other-diets-complete-comparison/

Weeks, C. (2019, February 13). *20 best foods to eat while intermittent fasting.* Eat This Not That; Eat This Not That. https://www.eatthis.com/intermittent-fasting-diet-foods/

Made in the USA
Middletown, DE
26 July 2022